W9-BTO-283

Welcome to the EVERYTHING® series!

These handy, accessible books give you all you need to tackle a difficult project, gain a new hobby, comprehend a fascinating topic, prepare for an exam, or even brush up on something you learned back in school but have since forgotten.

You can read an *EVERYTHING*® book from cover-to-cover or just pick out the information you want from our four useful boxes: e-facts, e-ssentials, e-alerts, and e-questions. We literally give you everything you need to know on the subject, but throw in a lot of fun stuff along the way, too.

We now have well over 100 *EVERYTHING*® books in print, spanning such wide-ranging topics as weddings, pregnancy, wine, learning guitar, one-pot cooking, managing people, and so much more. When you're done reading them all, you can finally say you know *EVERYTHING*®!

FACTS

Important sound bytes
of information

SSENTIALS

Quick handy tips

ALERT

Urgent warnings

QUESTIONS?

Solutions to
common problems

THE
EVERYTHING
Series

Dear Reader,

Congratulations! You're a parent! You will experience a wealth of joys over the next several years—your baby's first words, her hugs and kisses, and all the excitement of watching the life you created grow and flourish.

You have also made the healthy choice to give your baby the best start possible. Breastfeeding is truly an irreplaceable gift that only you can give to your child. Your milk is specially designed for your baby, and you have the ability to nourish and nurture your child the way nature intended.

As the parents of two breastfed children, we have experienced firsthand both the joys and the challenges of nursing. In addition to being a breastfeeding mother, Suzanne is a Certified Breastfeeding Educator and has seen the powerful benefits of breastfeeding time and time again.

We hope you enjoy this book, and we hope the knowledge you gain will empower you in your relationship with your health care providers.

Thank you for making the decision to breastfeed your baby. We feel privileged to be a part of your parenting experience.

Best wishes,

Suzanne Fredregill

Ray Fredregill

THE EVERYTHING BREASTFEEDING BOOK

Basic techniques and reassuring
advice every new mother
needs to know

Suzanne Fredregill
and Ray Fredregill

Adams Media Corporation
Avon, Massachusetts

EDITORIAL
Publishing Director: Gary M. Krebs
Managing Editor: Kate McBride
Copy Chief: Laura MacLaughlin
Acquisitions Editor: Bethany Brown
Development Editor: Christel A. Shea

PRODUCTION
Production Director: Susan Beale
Production Manager: Michelle Roy Kelly
Series Designer: Daria Perreault
Layout and Graphics: Brooke Camfield,
Colleen Cunningham, Michelle Roy Kelly,
Daria Perreault

An Everything® Series Book.
Everything® is a registered trademark of Adams Media Corporation.

Published by Adams Media Corporation
57 Littlefield Street, Avon, MA 02322 U.S.A.
www.adamsmedia.com

ISBN: 1-58062-582-7
Printed in the United States of America.

J I H G F E D C B A

Library of Congress Cataloging-in-Publication Data
Fredregill, Suzanne.
The everything breastfeeding book: basic techniques and reassuring advice
every new mother needs to know / by Suzanne and Ray Fredregill.
p.   cm.
Includes index.
ISBN 1-58062-582-7
1. Breastfeeding—Popular works. I. Fredregill, Ray. II. Title. III. Series.
RJ216 .F734   2002
649'.33—dc21   2002003794

This publication is designed to provide accurate and authoritative information with regard to the subject matter covered. It is sold with the understanding that the publisher is not engaged in rendering legal, accounting, or other professional advice. If legal advice or other expert assistance is required, the services of a competent professional person should be sought.
—From a *Declaration of Principles* jointly adopted by a Committee of the American Bar Association and a Committee of Publishers and Associations

Illustrations by Barry Littmann and Eulala Conner.

This book is available at quantity discounts for bulk purchases.
For information, call 1-800-872-5627.

Visit the entire Everything® series at everything.com

Contents

Dedication

To our breastfed children, Meaghan and Ian, and to our parents.

Introduction

Making a "decision" to breastfeed is really very new. Since long before recorded history, breastfeeding was the only choice women had. If a mother was unable to nurse her child, family or friends who were lactating would nurse the baby for her. In some cases, wet nurses were employed by the wealthy. A wet nurse was a lactating woman who was paid to nurse and care for another's child. She often nursed her young charges in addition to her own children.

Today, almost two and a half million women in the United States breastfeed their newborns. That's approximately 60 percent of all new mothers. The practice of breastfeeding instead of feeding an infant formula from a bottle is slowly gaining ground. It's a trend that health care professionals enthusiastically welcome. They know that "breast is best." Your breastfeeding relationship with your child will have far-reaching rewards for both you and your baby, as well as your entire family.

Nursing your child is a relaxing and enjoyable experience that just might be one of the most satisfying relationships you've ever had. There's nothing like the emotional closeness of breastfeeding. When your baby looks up at you adoringly and smiles, you'll know you've made the right choice.

Breastfed children have fewer infections, fewer digestive problems, and better brain development than formula-fed babies, and that's just the beginning. Breastfeeding also helps your body recover from labor and birth, and decreases your risk of breast cancer. There are even financial and environmental advantages. Breastfeeding your child is a responsible, loving, and natural choice.

However, although breastfeeding is natural, learning this new skill doesn't come naturally to everyone. Some women are lucky enough to experience only a few problems, but many need a little help at first. In the past, women grew up surrounded by breastfeeding friends and family members. Girls growing up during that period in history had the opportunity to learn the "womanly art" from their female role models. By the time they had children, they had seen and perhaps assisted with breastfeeding on many occasions. If they had a problem, they could consult with their mothers, female friends, or a midwife.

Things changed in the twentieth century. Bottle feeding of infant formulas became much more common than breastfeeding. Women were persuaded by both advertisers and the medical community that infant formula was at least as good as breastmilk, and certainly more convenient. Today, we know that nothing compares to breastmilk. Unfortunately, decades of bottle feeding have left most women without the social support and knowledge necessary for breastfeeding success. Now, we have to rely on a more formal method of breastfeeding education.

This book will provide you with techniques, tips, and insights that will enhance your breastfeeding experience. The information provided is based on current research and recommended best practices in the field of breastfeeding education.

You can breastfeed. There is no better nourishment for your baby than your own milk. Your milk is specially designed for your child whether premature or full term, infant or toddler. With a little preparation, practice, confidence, and patience, you'll be well on your way toward breastfeeding success.

CHAPTER 1

The Importance of Breastfeeding

Despite all the fantastic things humans have accomplished, we've never been able to come up with a better food than breastmilk for your baby. That's not to say we haven't tried! The formula options available can be mind-boggling. Luckily for us, the simplest choice is also the healthiest choice. No infant formula can meet your baby's needs the way your own breastmilk does.

Breastfeeding Is Good for Your Baby

Breastmilk is the elixir of life for your baby. Each precious drop gives her exactly what she needs in just the right amounts. It's an incredible mixture that's constantly changing to meet your baby's needs.

Digestibility

One of the greatest advantages of breastmilk is how easily your baby can digest it. This is especially important during the first year of life when your baby will be growing more rapidly than at any other time. Part of the reason breastmilk is so digestible is that the proteins are smaller than formula proteins. The vitamins and minerals in breastmilk are also more easily absorbed by your baby's body than those found in formula or other supplements. But breastmilk goes beyond just being easy to digest.

FACTS

Breastmilk is the best milk for your baby! The American Academy of Pediatrics (AAP); the World Health Organization (WHO); The Association of Women's Health, Obstetric and Neonatal Nursing (AWHONN); the Federation International of Gynecology & Obstetrics (FIGO); the International Confederation of Midwives (ICM); the International Lactation Consultant Association (ILCA); the Women, Infants, and Children Supplemental Program (WIC); and the U.S. Department of Health and Human Services all recommend exclusive breastfeeding for at least the first six months.

Enzymes in breastmilk work with your baby's digestive system to help her get the most out of every feeding. As a result, breastmilk goes through your baby's system twice as fast as formula while providing her with better nourishment than any other food source.

Yes, this means that your young, breastfed baby will have more frequent bowel movements than formula-fed babies of the same age. It also means your nursing baby will want to eat more frequently than a formula-fed baby. But, your baby will spit up less and have fewer cases of indigestion. Because breastfed infants generally eat smaller meals than formula-fed babies, there's less opportunity for spitting up.

The easy digestibility of breastmilk is also important in lessening the severity of gastroesophageal reflux (GER). GER is a heartburnlike pain that happens when stomach acids back up into your baby's esophagus. There's a circular muscle where the esophagus meets the stomach that normally prevents this from occurring. However, in some babies, it takes most of their first year of life for that muscle to develop properly.

If you've ever had acid reflux, just imagine having it as a baby. Like the old Leslie Gore song says, "You would cry, too, if it happened to you!"

Stools

As a direct result of breastmilk's digestibility, your baby's stools will be smaller, softer, and less likely to knock you out. No one is promising that diaper changing will be like a trip to the perfume counter, but with fewer fats and proteins passing through your baby's system undigested, the smell of stools is not just reduced, it's changed.

Keeping track of your baby's diapers is a good way to assess your milk production. Babies typically have at least eight to ten wet diapers and four to six stools per day when they are getting enough to eat.

Immunity

At birth and until approximately four months of age, your child's immune system is underdeveloped. All sorts of viruses, fungi, bacteria, and other villains will try to invade your baby's body. Without a mature immune system, she's an easy target. But, once again, it's breastmilk to the rescue!

Many of the ingredients in your breastmilk help fight infections or promote the growing strength of your baby's own immune system. Breastmilk contains ingredients that shield the intestines, help friendly bacteria grow, keep necessary iron away from the invading cells, and cut through the invaders' cell walls.

FACTS

An exciting study on breastmilk and immunology was featured in the June 1999, Discover magazine under the title "Got Cancer Killers?" A protein (dubbed "HAMLET") in breastmilk causes cancer cells to commit suicide. HAMLET is reportedly deadly to "every cancer we test it against," say the researchers. Imagine if a cancer cure has been literally under our noses all along!

Most amazingly, breastmilk is a living substance. Like blood, it's teeming with millions of disease-fighting cells called antibodies. These antibodies are nature's way of immunizing your baby against every disease you have ever been exposed to. And that protection constantly improves. If you are exposed to a new germ, your body will pass on immunity to that germ to your baby through your milk. "Breastmilk immunization" can happen before you even notice the first symptoms of illness.

Adults who were breastfed as infants have lower incidences of diabetes, Crohn's disease, and coronary heart disease. Furthermore, research finds that breastmilk kills germs in babies' mouths and helps heal mothers' cracked nipples. Some moms even put it on cuts and scrapes. It's like your immune system in an easy-to-use liquid.

Intelligence

Your baby's brain grows at a fantastic rate in those first few months. You won't always be able to tell as she lies in your arms looking so serene, but this is her brain's busiest developmental stage. Behind that cute brow, there's a firestorm of activity. Neural pathways are forming. With every moment, some paths are strengthened and others fade. Your baby needs the proper materials for this important work, and your breastmilk is a virtual grocery list of exactly those ingredients. Studies have found up to a 10-point IQ advantage in breastfed children.

Fats and sugars in your milk are custom-tailored for brain growth. Babies need fat for brain development for at least the first two years of their lives. The fats found in your breastmilk help form the insulation on the electrical wiring of your baby's brain, and they make your baby smarter, too.

Your milk is specially made for your baby, just as cow's milk is made for calves and goat's milk is made for baby goats. The types of proteins, fats, and other nutrients found in cow's milk are just what a baby cow needs, but your baby's needs are different. Your breastmilk will actually change as your baby grows. For example, your body produces less fat for older babies than for newborns, while premature infants receive breastmilk that's richer and higher in calories.

Colic

Colicky babies cry and fuss a lot. It's impossible to over-emphasize just how much. It is like an unending stomachache. While the exact causes are unknown, one thing remains true across the board: Babies with colic are unhappy. Mothers with colicky babies aren't exactly thrilled about it, either.

The good news is that babies who are exclusively breastfed have a much lower incidence of colic (although that's not to say it can't happen). Breastfeeding infants can be colicky. A newborn's digestive system might not be able to fully digest anything—even breastmilk. However, when breastfed babies are colicky, it's usually less severe and for a shorter period of time than it would be if they were getting formula.

Emotional State

Babies often fall asleep at the breast, full and content. Breastmilk contains ingredients that stimulate your baby's body to produce a hormone called cholecystokinin (CCK). CCK relaxes your baby and helps her sleep. It's the same hormone that makes you feel drowsy after a big meal.

The act of nursing is also comforting to your baby and satisfies her need to suck. The skin-to-skin contact keeps her warm. Your body temperature will actually adjust itself in response to hers. Nestled in your arms, she feels safe and secure. The closeness and intimacy of the feeding experience fosters your baby's sense of trust and makes it easier for her to communicate her needs to you. And you smell good, just like your milk.

The profound emotional connection you make with your baby grows into the connection you will have with your child. Nursing your baby makes you more in tune with her needs and feelings. She will feel secure and develop a trust in you that will serve as a strong foundation for her entire childhood.

Weight

Breastfed babies generally don't gain weight as quickly in the first few days as formula-fed babies, but they soon catch up. Many breastfeeding parents are concerned that their child seems underweight according to the doctor's charts. Don't let the growth chart worry you. Those weights are based on formula-fed infants, not breastfed babies. Formula-fed infants are overweight, while breastfed babies are leaner.

Formula and breastmilk generally average about the same number of calories per ounce. The difference is in the other ingredients and in the delivery system. Cow's milk is made to build body mass. The types of fats and proteins it contains encourage early weight gain. This makes sense for an animal that will gain hundreds of pounds in its first year of life. Breastmilk, on the other hand, contains a healthier balance of body and brain builders. It also changes as your baby suckles. At first, your baby gets the protein-rich foremilk. As she continues to nurse, your calorie-rich hindmilk lets down. With formula, she always gets the full-calorie version.

Facial Development

Babies suck differently on breasts than they do on bottles. The breast fills the mouth more completely. Breastfeeding works the entire mouth, while bottle feeding exercises only the front. The sucking movements affect babies' facial development. Breastfed babies tend to have larger nasal space and better jaw alignment, which means a reduced risk of snoring, sleep apnea, and orthodontic work later in life.

Allergies

Allergies are blamed for problems in children and adults, ranging from the classic hay fever all the way to behavioral difficulties. Infants are especially vulnerable to food allergies because of what some doctors call the leaky gut syndrome. The cells lining a baby's intestinal walls are just not packed together densely enough at birth to stop food proteins, or allergens, from entering the body.

FACTS

Colostrum is the yellowish fluid your breasts produce immediately following the birth of your baby. Many cultures have regarded colostrum as "dirty milk" and kept it from babies, but the truth is just the opposite: It's exactly what a newborn needs. Colostrum knocks out germs even more effectively than regular breastmilk and helps your baby get a healthy start in many other ways.

If you practice exclusive breastfeeding during your baby's first six months, you don't need to worry too much about food allergies. If you feed formula, however, you need to be aware of a host of potential allergens in the mix.

Breastmilk meets your baby's needs perfectly. It contains substances that help "seal the leaks" in your baby's intestinal lining while other substances help the lining to grow. Around six months of age, your baby's leaky intestinal lining achieves "closure." Babies becomes less sensitive to allergens and can start trying different foods.

Breastfeeding Is Good for You, Too

Not only is putting your baby to breast good for your baby, it's been shown time and again to have some impressive advantages for moms, too. You will experience short-term benefits such as delayed periods, as well as reduced risks of breast cancer and osteoporosis farther down the road.

Postpartum Recovery

If a doula or midwife assists your birth, she'll be sure your newborn breastfeeds in the first hour after delivery. Besides the fact that professional childbirth assistants nearly always advocate breastfeeding for baby, it's also an important part of your natural recovery from labor and delivery. Breastfeeding releases the hormone oxytocin, which causes your uterus to contract, thereby helping stop the flow of blood and delivering the placenta in one piece. If you choose not to breastfeed, your doctor will intervene with an injection of Pitocin, a synthetic form of oxytocin, to aid in the delivery of your placenta.

Amenorrhea

Amenorrhea is big word with a little definition: no periods. Many women enjoy time off from their menses for the first six months of breastfeeding. The benefits of this little break are more than just convenience.

Lactational amenorrhea (the pausing of your menstrual cycle while breastfeeding) means reduced fertility. As long as you are exclusively breastfeeding, you're much less likely to become pregnant. With lactational amenorrhea, women enjoy a 98 to 99 percent effective method of birth control. Best of all, it's completely natural.

Mother Nature's family planning: Six weeks of postpartum abstinence followed by six months of breastfeeding-induced amenorrhea gives you over sixteen months between births. However, amenorrhea is different for every woman. Sometimes the shortest separation from your baby can derail the process.

The other benefit of lactational amenorrhea is the prevention of anemia. Because breastfeeding removes iron from your body at a rate of about 0.3 milligrams per day, doctors have long considered it to be a cause of anemia in new mothers. As researcher Ted Greiner points out on his Web site, the amount of iron new moms would normally lose with their period is retained when their menses stop due to breastfeeding. In other words, instead of losing large amounts of iron to your period, you can lose much smaller amounts to your baby.

Traditionally, people have viewed breastfeeding as being a "draw" on the mother's body. Today, we know that it's just not true. Breastfeeding plays an important role in helping you recover from pregnancy and childbirth. Ample evidence exists that pregnancy can cause maternal anemia. Through breastfeeding, nature provides the remedy.

Cancer Prevention

You'll enjoy a significant reduction in your risk for breast cancer as a result of nursing your child. This protection has been found in women who have breastfed for as little as three months. The longer you nurse, the lower your risk of developing breast cancer. If you breastfeed for two years, you may cut your chances of breast cancer in half!

Other cancers are less likely in women who have breastfed, too. Ovarian, uterine, and cervical cancers are less common in women who have breastfed. No one is entirely certain how breastfeeding protects you from these potential killers, but one theory suggests that lactation's suppression of estrogen production plays an important role. Estrogen is a hormone that promotes cell growth in your reproductive anatomy and has been linked with female reproductive cancers. When you lactate, your body produces less estrogen. Lower levels of estrogen mean less growth. Less growth means less opportunity for cancers to develop.

Osteoporosis

You might have heard that pregnancy and breastfeeding deplete your body of calcium, leading to an increased risk of osteoporosis (brittle bones). The first part of that statement is true. Pregnancy and breastfeeding do use up your body's calcium reserve. But breastfeeding can actually help prevent osteoporosis. Here's how it works.

Weaning stimulates your body to increase bone density. Your postlactation bones will be stronger than they would have been if you had never breastfed at all. All you need to do is get enough calcium in your diet and your body takes care of the rest. Broccoli, almonds, whole wheat bread, oranges, peanut butter, dairy products, and beans are all calcium-rich foods.

Weight Loss

How would you like to eat more and still lose weight? When you breastfeed, your body will burn up the fat it stored during pregnancy to make milk. On top of that, you get to eat an additional 300 to 500 extra calories per day. You'll enjoy a good appetite and larger portions, and you'll lose pounds and inches.

Bonding

Nursing your little bundle of joy puts her close to you and gives you a chance to coo, cuddle, and take her in with all of your senses. We all talk about connecting with our children, and with breastfeeding the connection is real and physical. Skin-to-skin contact and suckling release powerful stress-reducing hormones (oxytocin and prolactin) in your body that relax you and give you a calm, pleasurable feeling. Those same hormones help you to literally fall in love with your newborn. Prolactin is sometimes called the "mothering hormone" because of the way it intensifies nurturing behavior.

If your blues extend beyond the first two weeks following the birth of your baby, you may be suffering from postpartum depression. If you find yourself feeling lethargic, have a loss of appetite, or have a hard time functioning, contact your doctor or midwife. You're not alone. Support is available.

Prolactin is also a natural tranquilizer. Within minutes of latch-on, you might begin to relax so much, you'll feel yourself getting sleepy. That's one of nature's little rewards.

Those same hormones also prevent the short-term feeling of sadness some women experience after childbirth. "Baby blues" results from the sudden drop in pregnancy hormones in your body after delivery. The baby blues can delay the bonding process and leave you unable to enjoy the first few days of motherhood. Breastfeeding signals your body to release the hormones that prevent those blues. If you breastfeed immediately following birth and wean gradually at a time of your choice, you can avoid the baby blues altogether.

Satisfaction

Breastfeeding can give you a strong sense of accomplishment, pride, and continuity with life and the world. You don't have to be an Earth Mother to appreciate the spiritual side of childbearing or your body's ability to feed your baby. Nursing is a powerful aspect of motherhood. Trusting your body to nourish your child is a deeply satisfying experience. Breastfeeding is a truly wonderful privilege.

Breastfeeding's Other Benefits

So, breastfeeding is good for your baby, and it's good for you. And in case that isn't enough to sell you, consider the secondary effects of going au naturel. No recycling, no late-night trips to the grocery store—and, best of all, breastmilk is free!

Environmental Convenience

Breastmilk isn't made in a factory or shipped to your local supermarket. No chemicals are used to manufacture colorful labels. You don't usually need a nonbiodegradable bottle or processed petrochemical nipple to use it. When you're done with a feeding, you don't have anything leftover to be hauled to the landfill. Maybe breastfeeding won't singlehandedly save the world, but then again, every little bit helps. After all, this is the world we'll be leaving to our children.

Formula needs to be prepared and heated. Those few extra seconds can seem like an eternity when your hungry baby is crying—especially in the middle of the night. With nursing, you don't have to worry about the quality of the water or the temperature of the milk. Breastmilk is the original convenience food.

Penny-Wise

Ka-ching! Breastfeeding will save you a significant chunk of change compared with feeding infant formula. If you choose bottle feeding, you can expect to spend over $1,200 annually on formula alone. If you mix that formula with store-bought water, add another $65 per year. Then you shell out more cash for the extra bottles, liners, nipples, and maybe even for dry cleaning to remove those formula-spitup stains.

One of the nicest things about breastfeeding is the convenience. The milk is always the perfect temperature, it's always clean, and you can't forget your breasts when you leave the house!

In addition, bottle-fed babies also keep the doctors busy. By the most conservative estimates, formula-fed babies run up over $200 more in medical expenses in their first year than breastfed babies do. They spend more time at the doctor's office because they're sick more than their breastfed friends.

Dads Love It!

Hey, new dads! As if having a happier, healthier family, a cleaner planet, and more money in your pocket wasn't enough, there's more! There are two often unspoken benefits to you that you might really appreciate: freedom from many feeding duties and an interesting new look to your already lovely partner. Breastfeeding is an experience the whole family can appreciate.

CHAPTER 2

Who Can Breastfeed?

The vast majority of mothers can successfully breastfeed. If you're able to give birth, you're almost certainly able to nurse your baby. There are exceptions, but they are uncommon and usually temporary. Most women who believe they were unable to breastfeed were probably just missing the two most important things every nursing mother really needs—confidence and support.

Breast Issues

The fact is that breast "issues" are most often a result of preconceived notions. In the past, a lack of information, education, and encouragement to breastfeed left many mothers making assumptions about why it wouldn't work for them. With the proper preparation and support, virtually all mothers can provide natural nourishment to their babies.

Breast Size

Breast size is mostly a matter of fat content, not milk-gland content. Small-chested women may actually have an advantage over their bustier friends when nursing low birthweight or premature babies. Very small babies sometimes find it difficult to latch onto an engorged breast. In those cases, smaller breasts can be an advantage.

QUESTIONS?

My nipples are pierced. Will the holes interfere with nursing?
Many women with pierced nipples have successfully breastfed. However, piercing of the nipples sometimes scars the milk ducts and inhibits the flow of milk. If your piercings have been infected or if you have multiple nipple piercings, you may find breastfeeding difficult. All jewelry must be removed before nursing.

If your breasts are large and you're self-conscious about their size, don't let that discourage you from breastfeeding, either. Large breasts don't generally get much larger with lactation. They also tend to leak less than smaller breasts.

There are advantages and disadvantages to different breast sizes, of course, but regardless of your size, stick with it, keep informed, and stay confident. You can have a successful breastfeeding experience.

Nipples

Like breasts, nipples come in a variety of types. There are nipples the size of champagne corks, nipples that hide inside the breast (inverted), and nipples that point up, down, or sideways. It's not unusual for a woman to have one nipple that's inverted and another that's not.

No matter what type of nipples you have, breastfeeding is possible. Inverted nipples can be coaxed out and large nipples can be worked around. Other moms have done it and you can, too.

Adoptive Moms

Yes, you can nurse your adopted baby! The process is not easy, but it can be done and has been done by many women. Your milk production can be started with the help of a breast pump and a little patience. However, initiating lactation without pregnancy requires a serious commitment.

A woman who produces milk for her own baby has the advantage of pregnancy. For nine months, her body has been preparing to feed a baby. Without those pregnancy hormones, you'll have to rely on manual stimulation as explained in detail in Chapter 12.

FACTS

The initiation of milk production is called "lactogenesis." There are new hormonal therapies being developed that can help a woman to lactate without pregnancy. However, these procedures may produce unpleasant side effects as well as the risk of unknown future complications. Check with your doctor.

Adoptive moms don't usually produce enough milk to fully feed a young infant, but don't let that discourage you. Nursing your baby isn't only about nutrition. Any amount of milk you produce is a precious gift for your child and the experience of nursing will be wonderful for both of you.

Drugs and Alcohol

The best practice when you're breastfeeding is to steer clear of all drugs, alcohol, and herbal products. Unfortunately, that way is blocked for some of us. Medical conditions or addictions can stand in the way of a drug-free lactation. If you smoke or drink, you'll need to make some changes during pregnancy and while nursing your child.

Medicine

The two main issues to consider before taking any medicine while breastfeeding are, Do the benefits to my health outweigh any risk to my baby? and, Do I need to wean my child to protect her from this medication? Some medications are harmless to your nursing infant. Others are less safe. Fortunately, permanent weaning is rarely necessary. Although many medicines will enter your milk supply, the amounts that reach your child are usually small. As a result, breastfeeding is compatible with a wide variety of pharmaceuticals.

Some medications are not safe to use while breastfeeding. If temporary weaning due to medication becomes necessary, it's important to use a breast pump to maintain your milk production. You'll need to "pump and dump" as often as your baby would nurse.

If you're taking a prescription drug on a doctor's order, remind your doctor that you plan to breastfeed. Some doctors routinely advise mothers to wean while medicated because they are not well informed about breastfeeding. It's often a good idea to talk to your pediatrician about prescriptions from other doctors. Your midwife or lactation consultant is also a good source of information.

While many drugs are considered safe for nursing moms, certain types are considered off-limits. Some of these drugs will affect your baby, while others can decrease your milk production. Some sources consider most medications to be off limits, while other sources consider the majority of medications to be compatible with breastfeeding.

It can be difficult to know whose advice to take. Doctors and drug companies both like to be on the safe side. If they don't have proof a particular drug is safe for breastfeeding, they recommend weaning. As a rule, you should be able to safely take any medicine your child can take and continue to nurse without worry. However, you should avoid combining medications if possible.

As your baby grows, it becomes safer for you to take medications. In the meantime, take the minimum amount necessary to ensure your comfort and health. A sick mom has a hard time taking care of her child. Sometimes, you have to take care of yourself first.

MEDICATIONS TO AVOID WHEN BREASTFEEDING

TYPE	COMMENTS
Acne products	Isotretinoin and tretinoin are unsafe when nursing. Other products are safe, but treated areas should not touch baby.
Antibacterials	Quinolones may cause damage to developing joints. Penicillins, while very safe, may cause diarrhea, thrush, or rash. Isoniazid has been linked to liver damage. Clindamycin can cause diarrhea and bloody stools. Chloramphenical may affect the taste of your milk. It has been linked to possible blood disorders in infants. Wean while using. Metronidazole requires weaning until twenty-four hours after last dose. Nitrofurantoin should be avoided with younger babies. Cephalosporins may cause allergic rash, diarrhea, and thrush.
Anticonvulsants	Most are safe, but valporic acid or carbamazepine may cause liver or blood damage.
Antidepressants	Most common effect on infants is drowsiness, but phenelzine and tranylcypromine should not be used.
Antifungal	Ketoconazole poses some risk of liver damage.
Antihistamines	May reduce milk flow and cause drowsiness and fussiness when taken in large amounts. Especially avoid cetirizine.
Anti-inflammatory	Ibuprofen is safe, but some others are unsafe for babies under ne year of age. Ketorolac, mefenamic acid, indomethacin may be toxic to nursing infants at any age.
Antiviral	Amantadine may decrease milk supply. Acyclovir is preferred.

MEDICATIONS TO AVOID WHEN BREASTFEEDING *(continued)*

TYPE	COMMENTS
Aspirin	Linked to Reye's syndrome and bleeding.
Chemotherapy	Very toxic, even in trace amounts.
Decongestants	Oral decongestants can cause fussiness. Sprays are better.
Diuretics	Most can suppress lactation.
Heart and blood pressure	Most seem safe, but acebutolol, atenolol, nadolol, sotalol, timolol may accumulate in baby's blood. Reserpine causes nasal stuffiness. Clonidine and guanfacine may reduce milk supply and accumulate in baby's body.
Hormones	Hormonal contraceptives can interfere with lactation if used in the first six weeks. DHEA may suppress lactation or affect infant. Estrogens can decrease your milk supply. Clomiphene can have serious effects on baby's sexual growth.
Lipid-Lowering drugs	May suppress necessary levels of cholesterol and inhibit brain and nervous system development.
Lithium	Can accumulate and cause lithium poisoning.
Narcotics	When given during labor, narcotics may inhibit lactation. They also cause drowsiness in nursing babies. Ergotamine may cause vomiting.
Pepto-Bismol	Salicylates can be toxic to nursing babies.
Postpartum	Ergonovine may suppress lactation.
Radioactive agents	Some may permanently affect your milk supply.
Sulfa drugs	Risk of jaundice.
Tetracycline	Linked to possible tooth staining. Some forms can color your milk.
Tranquilizers	May make baby sleepy, but generally safe except for clozapine, which can decrease white blood cell count.

Alcohol

While alcohol was advised against during your pregnancy, the rules for lactating moms are a little more lenient. A glass of wine with dinner or some champagne at a wedding is not completely out of the question. However, you need to be careful.

Alcohol does find its way into your milk. The negative effects for your baby include possible long-term immunity weakness and nervous system disorders. Infants in the first months of life are especially sensitive to alcohol's effects since their livers are not yet mature enough to eliminate it easily from their bloodstream. Older babies who rely less on mom for nursing and who have more body mass are better able to tolerate small amounts of alcohol in your breastmilk.

The good news is that alcohol clears from your breastmilk at about the same rate it clears from your bloodstream. If you have a single drink immediately after nursing, your milk should be alcohol-free by the time you nurse again in two to three hours (depending on your weight).

If your baby sleeps with you, your use of drugs or alcohol can be deadly. Normally, you sleep lightly when your child shares the bed. Parents "under the influence" are less aware. Every year there are cases where babies died because a parent rolled over and accidentally suffocated them.

Tradition maintains that an occasional serving of alcohol helps a mother produce more milk. Contrary to folk wisdom, however, alcohol appears to have a negative impact on successful breastfeeding. Studies have demonstrated a change in the taste and smell of breastmilk when mom drinks alcohol, and babies don't generally like it. Alcohol also reduces the levels of prolactin and oxytocin that are produced in your body when baby suckles. Prolactin aids in milk production as well as emotional bonding. Oxytocin plays a key role in your milk ejection, or letdown, response.

If you drink often, you may find your child weaning far earlier than you had planned. Your milk production, delivery, and flavor might lead to early weaning. On the other hand, an occasional drink seems relatively harmless if you allow it to clear from your bloodstream before nursing.

Smoking

If you haven't quit smoking already, this is a great time to stop. If you're a new parent, there are some important reasons to kick the habit. Smoking during pregnancy leads to low birthweight, reduced IQ, heart and lung difficulties for your baby, and an increased risk of complications following birth for both mother and child. After delivery, smoking continues to threaten your child's health.

If you nurse your baby and smoke, nicotine will find its way into your milk. Heavy smokers (more than a pack a day) may find their babies suffer from intestinal upsets and fussiness. Heavy smokers are also nearly twice as likely as nonsmokers to have colicky babies. Like alcohol, smoking has been linked to early weaning due to lowered milk production and inhibited letdown. However, research suggests that women who smoke less than a pack a day probably won't have any dangerous amounts of nicotine in their milk.

QUESTIONS?

Which smoking cessation product is best?
If you would like to quit smoking, the safest product to use is the nicotine patch. Nicotine levels in your blood are lower with the patch than they are with nicotine gum. If you choose gum, try to wait two to three hours before nursing.

Secondhand smoke is far more dangerous to babies than nicotine. Everyone needs to keep cigarette smoke far away from babies. Secondhand smoke has been linked to Sudden Infant Death Syndrome (SIDS) and respiratory infections. Just as you would insist on clean hands to hold your baby, insist on clean air for her, too. If Dad smokes, keeping smoke away from the baby is a great way to show he loves her.

The bottom line on smoking and breastfeeding is this: The benefits of breastfeeding generally outweigh the hazards of nicotine in your milk, but not those of secondhand smoke. If you can quit, congratulations! Your whole family wins. If you continue to smoke while nursing, you run a risk. At a minimum, try to cut down and keep the smoke away from your baby.

Controlled Substances

Like other drugs, controlled substances can interfere with your milk supply and letdown reflex. Marijuana, for instance, has been shown to reduce a mother's milk production by decreasing the level of prolactin she produces. It's also important to realize that any drugs you take can end up in your breastmilk, sometimes in a concentrated form. When you use, your baby uses. The damage done to a developing infant can be serious and permanent.

Street drugs like heroin and cocaine may be cut with harmful chemicals, and you can't be sure about their strength. Most importantly, recreational use of drugs impairs your ability to parent. Many drugs cause a loss of judgment and coordination. Good parenting takes a clear head.

If you have an addiction to a controlled substance, talk to your doctor about getting help.

Herbal Remedies

While it's always important to be careful, many herbs are safe for breastfeeding moms. There are herbs that can increase or decrease your milk supply. Others can take the place of regular, over-the-counter medications. If you choose to use herbal products, follow these guidelines:

❑ Check with your doctor.
❑ Use a brand that lists all active ingredients. The fewer ingredients, the better.
❑ Stick with a reputable brand.
❑ Check the expiration date.
❑ Bear in mind that herbal tinctures contain alcohol.

Herbs may seem natural and safe, but they are potent pharmacological substances. Many of the medicines found at the pharmacy are derived from herbs. Unlike commercial pharmaceuticals, however, herbal remedies and supplements aren't tested and approved by the FDA.

Multiple Births

Two babies? Now you know why you have two breasts! You can nurse twins or even triplets without worrying about your milk supply. Your breasts are marvelous, self-regulating milk production centers. The amount of milk they make is directly related to the amount of milk removed by a baby's suckling. More suckling equals more milk.

Caesarean Section

If you've delivered your child by Caesarean section, breastfeeding will help you to regain trust in your body's ability to mother while helping you to bond with your new baby. Sometimes, women who have delivered by C-section feel disappointed that their bodies have somehow failed them, but breastfeeding reinforces your confidence in your body's ability to nourish and nurture the new life you brought into the world.

Although C-section is major surgery, and your incision can be tender, your baby can nurse without causing stress on your sutures.

Mother's Medical Conditions

You may have a chronic health concern or condition, but that does not necessarily prevent you from breastfeeding successfully. Both your obstetrician (OB) and your pediatrician can give you information on the best way to accommodate your situation while providing the best feeding option for your baby.

Diabetes

Many diabetic mothers have successfully breastfed their children. Lactating can even help you control your blood sugar during the transition from pregnancy to postpartum. You'll need to pay close attention to your diet because lactating can seriously affect your blood sugar. Keep lots of water and snacks handy when nursing to help you avoid becoming hypoglycemic. Your regular insulin injections are safe for your nursing child. Unfortunately, oral hypoglycemic medications are not safe for you to use when breastfeeding. Discuss medication options with your doctor.

Diabetes will present you with some special challenges. Diabetic moms tend to get more yeast infections and suffer from mastitis more than nondiabetics. You'll need to give extra attention to your breasts and watch out for plugged milk ducts.

You're giving your baby a wonderful gift when you nurse. Best of all, breastfeeding your baby will help her to avoid becoming diabetic, too. Studies show that breastfed babies have a lowered incidence of Type 1 diabetes as well as fewer occurrences of obesity as adults.

HIV

The number of HIV-positive mothers with HIV-negative children is small, but the breastfeeding debate is huge. Some studies have found that the breastmilk of an infected woman can contain the HIV virus, but there is uncertainty about whether the virus detected is infectious. At this stage in the research, it's difficult to know what to do.

The AAP recommends that HIV-positive mothers in the United States use an alternate source of nutrition for their babies. On the other hand, many breastfeeding advocates believe that the risk of infection is so low and the benefits of breastfeeding so significant that everyone should breastfeed her baby. For mothers in extreme poverty or without access to safe drinking water, the protection breastfeeding offers a baby does seem to outweigh the chance of infection. For the rest of us, formula feeding is the more cautious route to take. In deciding to breastfeed, a woman with HIV should consider the possibility of transmitting the virus to her baby.

A woman with HIV is more likely to be infectious if she contracts the virus during the second trimester of pregnancy or later. Babies are most susceptible to HIV during the first few months of life. If you are HIV positive and decide to nurse, take extra care of your breasts. Your baby is more at risk if you're suffering from mastitis. Cracked and bleeding nipples, along with scrapes or cuts in your baby's lips, mouth, or throat, can also result in HIV transmission.

FACTS

If you're an HIV-positive mother with an HIV-positive child, breastfeeding will help your baby to stay healthy. Several recent studies have concluded that the immunity-enhancing qualities of breastmilk combat HIV in a baby's body.

HIV-infected women who take the drug AZT are much less likely to transmit HIV to their babies, either through birth or breastfeeding, although it does happen. If HIV turns into AIDS, breastfeeding is no longer an option. The risk of infection is simply too great.

Herpes

Herpes can be deadly to newborns if a mother contracts it during the last trimester of pregnancy. If you become infected at that time, a C-section might be your only option. Herpes on a woman's breast is less of a threat. With a few precautions, you can safely nurse your baby.

If you develop a herpes sore on your nipple, it's best not to let your baby nurse from that side until it's healed. Use a pump on the affected breast to maintain your milk supply. If the sore is somewhere else on your breast, cover it with a bandage or pad and continue to nurse as usual. Anytime you have an active outbreak of herpes, whether genital or oral (cold sores), you should take extra precautions. Wash your hands before handling your baby or your breasts and always keep your child away from herpes sores.

Cancer

A diagnosis of cancer doesn't mean it's time to wean. Babies cannot catch cancer through breastmilk and many cancer treatments are compatible with breastfeeding. If you are determined, you can continue to nurse your child despite biopsies or even more involved surgeries. However, there are some treatments that can affect your ability to breastfeed. With any type of cancer, it's important that you discuss your desire to breastfeed with your doctor and follow her advice.

ALERT

Tuberculosis is usually spread by adults with active TB, and children under the age of five have the greatest risk of infection. Mothers with untreated, active tuberculosis should not breastfeed their babies.

If your cancer treatment involves chemotherapy or the injection of radioactive compounds, you must wean your baby until those substances have left your body. Some radioactive agents remain in your body for many months. Chemotherapy drugs are among the most toxic medicines used. They will enter your breastmilk, and even a tiny amount can be harmful to your child. If you plan to resume nursing, you should pump and dump your milk until your doctor gives you the "all clear" sign.

Breast Surgeries

If you've had breast surgery, talk with your doctor about the possibility of breastfeeding your child. You might be pleasantly surprised. If it turns out that you are unable to produce enough milk for exclusive breastfeeding, don't be discouraged. Whatever amount of milk you can produce for your baby is wonderful. Every little bit contains the antibodies and nutrients that only you can provide. Remember, too, that nursing your baby isn't only about the milk. Breastfeeding is a special and loving time with your baby. If you want to nurse your child, you can purchase a supplemental feeding system. These devices allow your baby to nurse from your breast while receiving formula through tiny tubes. Another choice is to simply bottle feed formula after each nursing session.

Breast Reduction

Most women who have had breast reduction surgery can still produce some amount of milk. However, this type of surgery typically leaves women unable to produce enough milk to exclusively nurse their babies. In some reductions, the nipple is completely removed from the breast and reattached in a new location. If the nipples were completely severed, and are numb, breastfeeding is not possible. In some rare cases, severed nerves have actually grown back after breast reduction surgery, but this is very unusual.

Breast Augmentation

Breast augmentation surgery will not usually interfere with a woman's ability to produce milk. Most surgeons make the incisions near the armpit or under the fold of the breast. With the nipple left undisturbed, nursing is generally unaffected. Some new mothers worry about implant leakage into their milk supply, but there's no need to let that bother you. The fears about leaking implants that were all over the news a few years ago have turned out to be unsupported by any valid research. Whether your implants are silicone or saline, your milk is safe for your baby.

Baby's Medical Conditions

Although you may be in excellent health, it is possible that one of several infant conditions will present challenges for your breastfeeding plans. While most hospitals routinely screen newborns for a host of disorders, it is important that you notify your doctor if you have a family history of galactosemia, PKU, or any other hereditary conditions. A hospital lactation consultant is often available to guide you through these and other situations.

Jaundice

Jaundice is a condition that affects many newborns to some extent. Jaundiced babies appear yellow or orange because of an excess of bilirubin, a substance produced when a baby's body breaks down extra red blood cells. Jaundiced babies are often sleepy and need to be awakened to nurse. Normal newborn jaundice occurs within the first week of life and lasts no more than two weeks. Other types of jaundice may be due to medical conditions that require more advanced treatment.

If your baby is jaundiced, nursing him will help. Bilirubin leaves your child's body through his stools. Frequent nursings at the breast help your baby have frequent stools and eliminate excess bilirubin as quickly as possible.

Premature Birth

Preemies have special needs. They are usually very small and more susceptible to infections. They also suckle less effectively than full-term babies. To complicate breastfeeding even further, premature babies might need to be placed in the Neonatal Intensive Care Unit (NICU). With IVs and other medical procedures, nursing might not be possible.

Many parents feel helpless when their baby needs so much medical attention, but only a mother can provide her baby with the perfect food. Your breastmilk is exactly formulated for your child, whether the baby is premature or full term. Refer to Chapter 7 for alternative feeding methods. Pumping will help you feel connected with your child, even when you're unable to hold her; it will also keep your milk supply up for the day she's able to nurse.

Galactosemia

Galactosemia is a rare, inherited disorder that affects about 1 in every 60,000 newborns. Babies suffering from galactosemia are unable to process galactose, one of the simple sugars formed by the digestion of the milk sugar lactose. There may be no indication of a problem when the baby first nurses. Galactosemia is only diagnosable through newborn screening. Eventually, the galactose builds up to dangerous levels.

Damage to the liver, central nervous system, eyes, and kidneys can occur. Babies with galactosemia should never be fed breastmilk or ordinary infant formulas. Your pediatrician will recommend a special diet.

Because galactosemia is a recessive genetic trait, both parents can carry the gene without any symptoms. If anyone in your family has a history of galactosemia, tell your doctor immediately. Your doctor might recommend genetic counseling before pregnancy or delivery. Newborns are routinely checked in most states for galactosemia with a simple blood test. Make sure your child is tested.

Kari gave birth to her long-awaited daughter just before Thanksgiving. Lauren was born with meconium stain and was suctioned with a tube to clear her throat. She was slow to nurse, but suctioning, coupled with newborn jaundice, was thought to be the cause. They were released from the hospital Thanksgiving Day, after the standard newborn heel-stick.

QUESTIONS?

What is a meconium stain?
Meconium is your baby's first stool. It consists of swallowed amniotic fluid and excess cellular matter. Usually babies pass meconium after birth. However, sometimes meconium is passed inutero and can be inhaled by the baby, causing respiratory distress.

Because Lauren had lost 10 percent of her birthweight, Kari was determined to nurse. With the assistance of a lactation consultant and the support of a wonderful pediatrician, Kari expressed her milk and finger fed her baby. Lauren began to gain weight, but just as she was learning to feed at the breast, Kari received an urgent call from her doctor.

Eight days after birth, Lauren was identified through newborn screening to be presumptively positive for galactosemia. Ordinarily, the test results would have been back within two days. Because of the holiday weekend, it took six.

Until further testing could be completed, Lauren was put on a soy formula. For several weeks Kari expressed and froze her milk in the event that breastfeeding could continue. However, further testing confirmed that Lauren was galactosemic.

Kari has become an advocate for families affected by galactosemia. Lauren continues to thrive under her parents' informed and loving care.

PKU

Phenylketonuria (PKU) is a genetic condition found in 1 in every 16,000 newborns. Babies with PKU are unable to produce an enzyme that allows their bodies to absorb the amino acid phenylalanine. Dangerous levels of phenylalanine can build up in a PKU baby's body, causing symptoms ranging from rashes to central nervous system damage.

FACTS

Blood tests for phenylketonuria (PKU) and hypothyroidism are the only tests required by law in every state. Most states also require vitamin K injections, some form of eye care, and testing for galactosemia. Tests for jaundice, hypoglycemia, and sickle cell anemia are generally only performed when medically indicated. Be certain to tell hospital staff if you have a family history of any of these conditions.

Babies with PKU require frequent monitoring of their amino acid levels. They need just enough phenylalanine for growth, but an excess can be toxic. Breastmilk contains lower levels of phenylalanine than regular formula but is still not safe for exclusive feeding of a PKU baby. However, a combination of breastfeeding and a special infant formula is possible for these infants. Under a dietitian's supervision, you may be able to breastfeed a little bit every day.

If you have PKU and are pregnant, you need to pay close attention to your diet. Even if your baby doesn't inherit the condition, high levels of phenylalanine in your blood can cause serious harm to your unborn child.

CHAPTER 3

Breasts and Milk Production

You have the incredible ability to nourish your child exclusively from your own body for the first six months of his or her life. Lactation is an amazing gift that benefits both you and your baby in many ways. Although you don't necessarily need to know how the process works to be a successful breast-feeding mom, you might be surprised at just how miraculous the process of lactation is.

Breast Development

Breast buds begin developing in female embryos just four weeks after conception. By the time of birth, basic breast development is complete. The nipples, areolas, and even some milk ducts are in place along with a small pad of fat. Everything is functional on a very small scale.

From just after birth until puberty, breast development is almost on hold. Some milk ducts and glandular tissue grow, but the process doesn't really take off until ten to fourteen years of age.

FACTS

Some babies leak breastmilk at birth. In the past, people called it "witches' milk." Far from being some kind of unnatural event, such leakage is normal and not uncommon. The pregnancy hormones in your body that prepare you for lactation can also cause your newborn's breasts to produce milk. The hormones typically leave the baby's body in a few days and the symptoms pass.

At the onset of puberty, a hormone called estrogen is secreted by the ovaries, bringing about a rush of breast development. The mammary fat pad increases in size and the milk ducts grow longer and branch out. When the menstrual cycle begins, the hormone progesterone causes the development of breast alveoli, the milk producing cells.

By the age of twenty, the process is nearly complete. However, breasts actually continue to mature until either pregnancy or age thirty to thirty-five. Some women may wonder why, with all this growth, their breasts aren't larger. The important thing to remember is that breast development is your body's way of preparing you to nourish a baby. The size of your breasts does not affect your ability to produce milk. Breast size is actually determined by heredity and body fat, and has very little to do with your ability to nurse.

Childbirth naturally completes the cycle of breast development.

Breast Anatomy

A basic knowledge of breast anatomy is helpful in understanding milk production. Think of your lactating breasts as a kind of fruit salad. It sounds weird, but it will make sense in a minute.

The insides of your breasts are divided into sections like the inside of a grapefruit. Each of these sections is called a lobe. Every breast has fifteen to twenty-five lobes. Inside each lobe are twenty to forty smaller sections called lobules. The lobules contain the glands that produce milk. Those glands are called alvoli and they cluster together like grapes around the milk ducts. The milk ducts join together like grape stems and connect to the milk sinuses located under the areola.

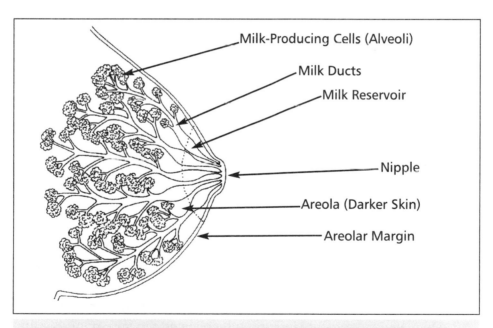

FIGURE 3-1: Internal Organization. The clusters of alveoli produce milk and the ducts transport it to the sinuses, where your breastmilk is stored until your baby's next feeding.

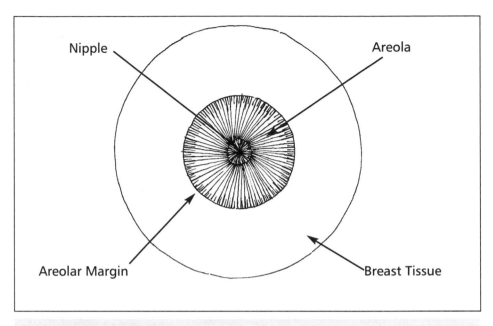

Nipple

Areola

Areolar Margin

Breast Tissue

FIGURE 3-2: External Diagram. The breast is divided into three sections. The areola is key to successful breastfeeding.

Your Changing Breasts

With the onset of your first pregnancy, your breasts get their marching orders. The placenta stimulates your body to produce hormones (estrogen and progesterone) that prepare your breasts for lactation. Recent animal research indicates that the placenta itself may actually produce those hormones. Your body responds to this wake-up call in several ways.

First, your nipples and areolas darken. This helps them to stand out from the surrounding tissue and act as a visual bull's-eye for your baby. Dramatic experiments in Europe highlighted the importance of the areola's darkening. After delivery, babies were placed face-down on their mother's abdomen. Amazingly, those little newborns zeroed in on their mother's nipples, crawled up, and latched onto a breast without any direction or assistance. All that from an infant who wouldn't know how to control her own body for months yet. This incredible inborn ability disappears soon after a baby's first hour of life.

Second, your breasts grow larger and sometimes tender. Throughout pregnancy, some women gain well over one and a half pounds in each breast as glandular tissue is being added to enable lactation. These milk-producing cells will replace a large portion of the fat cells in your breasts.

Third, your milk ducts grow. These ducts are the paths milk takes from the dairy in the alveoli to the sinuses under your areolas. Your breasts are doing road construction during pregnancy, increasing both the number of ducts and their size.

Finally, your Montgomery glands become noticeable as bumps on your areolas. These glands produce an oily substance that cleans and lubricates your nipples.

Studies indicate that women who have been pregnant enjoy a decreased risk of breast cancer compared to women who have never been pregnant. These findings imply that your breasts are just like the rest of your body in one important way—they are healthier when used the way nature intended.

At some point in your second trimester, the work is done and your breasts are ready to nourish your baby. The high levels of progesterone in your body prevent lactation from occurring before birth, but you may notice a fluid leaking from your breasts. This fluid is called colostrum and it varies from thin and clear to thick and white. Colostrum is formed when the cells inside your new milk glands dissolve. Some women leak a little colostrum during pregnancy and others don't—either case is perfectly normal.

How Your Breasts Produce Milk

Breasts are not like bottles; they aren't just containers for milk. Your breasts are never empty and you don't need to wait until you feel full to nurse. Milk is manufactured constantly, as long as there is demand. Milk production, or lactogenesis, normally begins with the birth of your baby. Labor and delivery start a physiological chain reaction. The expulsion of your placenta causes the levels of the hormones estrogen and progesterone in your body to fall. At the same time, nerve impulses from the uterus travel to the brain's hypothalamus gland. The brain then signals the pituitary gland to release the hormones prolactin and oxytocin.

Extra blood is sent to your breasts so they can start manufacturing milk. It's this extra blood, along with your milk coming in, that combine to engorge your breasts, sometimes painfully.

The prolactin released by your pituitary gland causes the grapelike clusters of alveoli to produce milk. The other hormone, oxytocin, aids in the ejection of milk from the breast.

It usually takes about seventy-two hours for your breasts to begin producing abundant milk. The process is completely under way within five days. During the first day or two of his life, your baby is nourished not with milk, but with your colostrum, the ideal first food for your infant.

Although your milk will come in after birth whether your child nurses or not, only the constant removal of milk from the breast can maintain milk production once you begin to lactate. Your baby's suckling signals your pituitary gland to release more oxytocin and prolactin. Just like in the beginning, these hormones cause your breasts to produce milk. If your baby drinks less milk than your breast produces, the excess milk remaining in your breasts will reduce future milk production.

It's a wonderfully self-regulating system. The more your child nurses, the more milk you produce. The less your child nurses, the less milk you produce. So, if you're worried about your milk supply, the solution is simply to nurse more often. Allowing your baby to nurse whenever she wants is also the best way to increase your milk supply. Supplementing breastmilk with formula short-circuits the whole process. Anything that reduces your baby's hunger or her need to suck will ultimately reduce your milk supply. That's why glucose, water, formula, and even pacifiers are not recommended for breastfeeding babies. Your baby needs to be hungry and eager to suckle when you put her to breast.

greater weight. After about a month, preterm milk changes into mature milk. Your body's ability to formulate the right quality of milk for your baby is nothing short of amazing.

Transitional Milk

Transitional milk is the mixture of colostrum and mature milk your breasts produce between birth and the time your mature milk comes in. Transitional milk still has an extra advantage to it because of its colostrum content. As time passes, it gives way to your mature milk.

Mature Milk

Mature milk begins to come in within seventy-two hours of birth and normally replaces transitional milk completely within five days postpartum. Your mature breastmilk will exclusively provide your baby with all of her nutritional needs for the first six months of life. Mature breastmilk is actually more than a single substance. Your baby receives two types of milk at each feeding, foremilk and hindmilk.

Foremilk

Foremilk is the milk that collects in the breast between feedings. About one third of the milk your baby drinks at each feeding will be foremilk. It's the first course of your baby's meal. Foremilk satisfies her need for water and energy. It's like a quick pick-me-up but it doesn't contain everything a growing baby needs. For a complete feeding, your baby needs to nurse long enough on one breast to get the hindmilk.

Hindmilk

Hindmilk is the main course. It's rich in nutrients and fats. Your baby needs both of those to grow. Almost two thirds of the human brain is composed of fat. Brain and nervous system development depends on fat, and your hindmilk delivers it. The richness of hindmilk also gives your baby a satisfied, full feeling that helps her know she's had enough to eat.

Breastmilk Contents

You might wonder what's so special about breastmilk. Actually, there are hundreds of ingredients identified in breastmilk that are missing from infant formula. Other ingredients are found in different concentrations. Human milk is unique and cannot be duplicated. Its ingredients have been tailored by millions of years of evolution to help human babies survive. However, even if every ingredient in human milk could be duplicated, breastmilk would still have significant advantages over formula.

Remarkably, your milk is alive. It's almost more like white blood than milk. Like blood, your milk is rich in antibodies that fight infections in your baby. Living cells from your body, called macrophages, enter your child's body through breastfeeding. These macrophages cruise through your baby's system gobbling up germs, which is especially important during the first months of life when your baby's own immune system is weak.

Your own milk also contains living enzymes that help your baby digest her meal. Formula can't do that. Neither can the cows' milk most formulas are based on. Of the hundreds of different kinds of animal milks, only human breastmilk is perfectly suited for human babies.

A PARTIAL COMPARISON OF HUMAN MILK AND COWS' MILK		
Carbohydrates	lactose	breastmilk has almost twice as much as cows' milk
	oligosaccharides	twelve times as much as cows' milk
Proteins	caseins	less than one tenth the amount of cows' milk
	lactalbumin	twice as much as cows' milk
	lactoferrin	present in human milk, but only trace amounts in cows' milk
	secretory immunoglobulin A (IgA)	seventy times as much as cows' milk
	lactoglobulin	none in human milk, but present in cows' milk; can lead to dietary protein allergy
Minerals	sodium, potassium, & magnesium	one third the amount of cows' milk
	chloride	half as much as cows' milk
	calcium	one quarter the amount of cows' milk

Human breastmilk is rich in the carbohydrates needed to fuel your child's active body and brain. Up to 40 percent of the calories in human milk comes from the milk sugar lactose. Human milk gets more of its energy content from lactose than any other animal milk. Lactose gives your milk a sweet taste and won't cause diarrhea like the processed sugars in formula might.

Baby-Friendly Food

The proteins in human milk are also friendlier to your baby's digestive system. Most of the protein in cows' milk is in the form of casein, which forms hard curds in your baby's stomach. Breastmilk proteins are more easily absorbed and put less of a strain on your baby's system. One protein, immunoglobulin A, seals your baby's intestinal tract against allergens and infections. Another, lactoferrin, keeps iron away from the germs in your baby's body so they can't use it to reproduce.

The protein in our food is broken down by digestion into compounds called amino acids. Amino acids are the building blocks used to construct and maintain your body. Breastmilk contains ideal levels of taurine, an amino acid that builds and maintains the brain and eyes. Human milk also contains just the right levels of phenylalanine and tyrosine. Cows' milk and formula have too much. Excessive amounts of these two amino acids can lead to a serious medical condition called PKU in infants.

FACTS

Amino acids build cells, form antibodies, carry oxygen, aid in cell reproduction and muscle operation, and perform many other tasks in the human body. There are twenty-two known amino acids. Eight cannot be manufactured in the body. Those eight are called the essential amino acids and must come from dietary sources. Milk, cheese, eggs, and meat are good sources of the essential amino acids for a breastfeeding mother.

Another vital ingredient in infant nutrition is fat. Fats and cholesterol are especially important to your baby's brain and nervous system

development, and your breastmilk has all he needs. Human milk is your baby's only source for the important brain-builder docosahexaenoic acid (DHA). Breastmilk is also low in saturated fats and high in polyunsaturated fats. Polyunsaturated fats help build brain and nerve cells. Saturated fats only help body growth. Research suggests that adequate levels of the right dietary fats might even help reduce your child's risk of developing diseases like multiple sclerosis.

The balance of nutrients is also important. The mix of minerals and vitamins in human milk is carefully proportioned for human babies. An excess of any one vitamin or mineral can affect the body's absorption of other nutrients or encourage harmful bacteria to grow. Breastmilk provides nutrients in both a form and an amount your child's body can easily use.

Nature designed the breastfeeding mechanisms so well that they respond to your baby's changing dietary needs. At different times in your baby's life and even at different moments during a feeding, the composition of your milk changes.

Colostrum

Colostrum is the first milk your breasts produce. It's powerful stuff and just what your newborn needs. Colostrum contains more protein, minerals, salt, vitamin A, nitrogen, white blood cells, and antibodies than mature milk. It's also lower in fat and sugar. Frequent feedings of colostrum help your baby get off to a great start. You'll produce about two tablespoons of colostrum in the first twenty-four hours after birth. That's just the right amount for your baby's tiny tummy. In addition to the nutritional benefits, colostrum also helps clean the meconium from your newborn's intestines. Meconium causes your baby's stools to have the appearance and consistency of tar. It's a natural occurrence, but one th we're all happy to see end. The speedy elimination of meconium redu the risk of jaundice in your newborn.

Preterm Milk

Preterm milk is produced if you give birth to a premature child milk is high in fats, proteins, and sugars to help your baby grow a

Foremilk and hindmilk work together to custom-tailor the breastfeeding experience throughout your lactation. When your baby isn't really hungry but wants to nurse for emotional closeness, she receives only low-fat foremilk. The same is true for older babies who nurse less frequently.

Milk Ejection Reflex or Letdown

The release of milk caused by oxytocin is called the letdown reflex or the milk ejection reflex. When your baby suckles, the stimulation to the nipple signals your body to release oxytocin, the hormone responsible for milk ejection. The oxytocin reaches your breast tissue where it causes the tiny muscles surrounding the milk-producing glands to contract. The milk is forced down the milk ducts to the sinuses beneath your areolas. When your baby nurses, she compresses the milk sinuses and the milk is pushed through the holes in your nipple.

It takes a few moments after the start of nursing for letdown to occur. Fifty percent of women will know the moment it happens and 50 percent won't. You might feel a tingling in your breasts or even a "pins and needles" sensation. That feeling is followed by a sudden release of milk. Some women will experience multiple milk ejection reflexes during a single feeding. Sometimes, letdown occurs when you are away from your baby. When that happens, milk can shoot out in streams. Major tip: Nursing pads—don't leave home without them!

ESSENTIALS

Oxytocin production can be easily influenced by your state of mind. If you're stressed or distracted, your letdown reflex might be delayed or inhibited. Other factors that might affect letdown include cold, pain, fatigue, caffeine, and nicotine. Fortunately, the prolactin you produce when baby suckles is a natural tranquilizer.

Once you have letdown, you'll feel thirsty, relaxed, and drowsy. You'll also feel your uterus contract. This is sometimes referred to as "afterpains." They will decrease in intensity with time.

With letdown, you might notice your milk flowing faster and your baby swallowing more frequently. Even if you can't feel it, if you can see and hear your baby swallow, you'll know it's happened.

Often in the morning, when milk is most abundant, your infant may gag or cough. You can decrease the flow of milk by altering positions.

Breast and Nipple Care

Your breast is almost like a self-cleaning oven. The Montgomery glands surrounding your nipples secrete an oily substance that keeps your breasts clean and moist. There is very little you need to do. In fact, overzealous cleansing of your nipples can lead to problems. Soap will dry your nipple and can cause painful cracking. Soap also leaves unpleasant-tasting residue on your skin.

When bathing, use plain water to wash your breasts and nipples. If you wash your hands before and after each feeding, your breasts will stay clean. After nursing, rub some breastmilk over your areola. Your milk has medicinal properties that will help keep your nipple healthy. Then, if possible, let your nipples air dry.

SSENTIALS

Use plain water when washing your breasts. Avoid soaps and gels, even in the shower. Your nipples produce natural oils that cleanse and moisturize the areola. Soap will remove these oils and can cause problems for nursing.

If you wear nursing pads, change them often. The warm, dark, and wet pad is an ideal breeding ground for germs. The best pads are washable, breathable cotton. Nursing pads with waterproof liners only hold the moisture in.

CHAPTER 4

Prenatal Preparation

Forewarned is forearmed (and you'll wish you had four arms!). Try to take advantage of the free time you enjoy now to get prepared for parenting your newborn. Fortunately, there are lots of things you can do now to make breastfeeding more successful and less stressful. Now is the time to toe up to that starting line and get set to go. You'll be glad you did.

Nipple Assessment

One of the first steps toward breastfeeding success is determining your nipple type. You can do this by conducting a nipple self-assessment. Roll your nipple between your fingers, have your partner stimulate your breasts, or open the freezer and stand in the cold air. How do your nipples react? Every nipple is different, even when they're on the same person. Regardless of your nipple type, you can still breastfeed.

Inverted Nipples

Nipples become inverted due to tight connective tissue bands under the areola. Inverted nipples appear to dent inward. (Flat nipples are caused by the same restrictive bands.) Both of these nipple types make it difficult for babies to latch on. It's still possible to breastfeed, but it might take a little extra effort. You can safely evert your nipples under the guidance of your lactation consultant. One of two methods will usually draw them out.

FIGURE 4-1:
Breast shell

FIGURE 4-2:
Hoffman's Technique

Breast shells—Breast shells are a wonderful invention for mothers who want to nurse but have inverted or flat nipples. They look like little dome-shaped cups with holes in the middle. Breast shells are worn inside your bra and fit over the nipple to put gentle pressure on the breast's connective bands and push the nipple out and through the opening. Other holes provide ventilation to keep your nipples dry.

You can wear shells during the last trimester of your pregnancy for a couple of hours per day. Then, gradually increase to approximately ten hours at a time. Once your baby is born, you can continue to use them. Breast shells don't hurt and no one can tell you're wearing them. They also come in handy if you have sore nipples.

Hoffman's Technique—Another method used by midwives and lactation consultants is called Hoffman's Technique. Hoffman's helps stretch the base of the nipple and gives your baby a more pliable area to latch onto. To practice this technique, place your thumbs on each side of your nipple and while gently pressing inward, pull your thumbs away from each other in a stroking motion. Now position your thumbs near the top and bottom of your nipple and repeat. You can do this several times each day during the last trimester. Ask your doctor or midwife to demonstrate this maneuver on your next OB visit.

Breast pumps—After your baby is born, you can use the suction of a breast pump to pull your nipple out just prior to putting baby to the breast, but only for as long as it takes to get the nipple erect. You need to use the pump only on the side baby has difficulty latching onto. Remember, he is feeding from the breast, not the nipple, but he must be able to extend the nipple to the back of his throat. Any breastmilk expressed by the pump can be saved for later use.

Some women with flat or inverted nipples are able to feed without any nipple preparation at all. Often, your baby will provide the best suction and the problem will take care of itself.

Nipple Preparation

It was once believed that nipples must be "toughened" to prepare for nursing. This is no longer considered best practice. Research has found that the cause of sore nipples isn't nursing friction. It's poor latch. In other words, the problem is how your baby takes the nipple into his mouth. When your baby latches onto your breast correctly, your nipples won't hurt.

The only thing you really need to do to prepare yourself for breastfeeding is become familiar with your breasts. You might not be comfortable with this at first. Women are taught to be self-conscious about their bodies from childhood, and often feel embarrassed about the size and shape of their breasts. Not only do they wear bras to support the weight of their breasts, they sometimes wear them just to keep their breasts covered.

Don't overstimulate your nipples during these self-assessment techniques! Nipple stimulation during pregnancy can cause uterine contractions and, potentially, premature labor. STOP if you feel any contractions. If contractions do not subside, contact your health care provider.

Our society has been so successful in sexualizing breasts that we have come to believe they are purely sexual organs. Getting to know your breasts is education, not masturbation. This kind of self-exam is not unlike what women do to screen for breast cancer. All you have to do is give your breasts a mere fraction of the attention that your partner gives them and you'll learn everything you need to know. Then, you'll feel comfortable and confident that these self-regulating wonders will provide ample nourishment for you baby.

Social-Emotional Preparation

Getting physically ready for your newborn is only the beginning. It's equally important to prepare yourself emotionally for this event that will change your life forever. Once your baby arrives, life as you know it is over. For the next year or more, you will truly understand the term "joined at the hip." With time, you'll wonder what life was like BC (Before Children). You will fall in love all over again and want to provide the very best life has to offer for your new baby.

You've also made the commitment to breastfeed. What will this mean for you? Will you return to work in six weeks? Will you stay home and exclusively nurse your baby? Now is the time to think about how breastfeeding will impact these decisions and your life.

If you are of low or middle income, contact your WIC program, United Way, or Visiting Nurse Services organization for additional assistance.

If you're going back to work, think about where you will express your milk. Talk to your employer about policies that support breastfeeding mothers. Seek out child care providers who are breastfeeding-friendly and who will allow you to stop by for an afternoon feeding or at the very least provide your baby with your expressed milk. Talk to other nursing mothers about techniques they've used and have them share their stories with you. Call a lactation consultant and schedule an appointment before your baby arrives. Search the Web for breastfeeding sites that offer the latest research. Find out what classes are offered within your community or join a breastfeeding mothers' group like La Leche League.

Begin to think of yourself as a breastfeeding parent!

Breastfeeding Supplies

At some point during your last trimester, your friends and family might hold a baby shower for you. In addition to Onesies, bibs, rattles, blankets, and a car seat, the items listed below would be great to have on your wish list.

Bras

When you head to the mall to buy a couple of comfortable nursing bras, you'll sigh as you pass Victoria's Secret, wondering why they didn't pick up on this marketing opportunity. Then you'll head right to the granny bra section of the nearest department store. There are several styles to choose from, but your goal is to find a comfortable bra that supports your enlarged breasts and is easy to operate. Here are a few factors to take into consideration:

FIGURE 4-3:
Nursing Bra

- Your cup size and bra (band) size will increase during pregnancy and will change when you nurse. You can expect to increase at least one size in each of these areas over the next couple of weeks.

- You'll be using the one-handed draw method for the next several months, so you'll need a bra that opens from the top to release the flap. Your new bra should also have adjustable straps, be easily breast-accessible, and refasten in a single smooth swoop. With time, you'll be able to maneuver your bra blindfolded, which is what you'll be doing when you nurse in public.

- Comfort and support are crucial. Your bra should support not only your breasts, but part of your underarm. Your breast tissue extends beyond the obvious. Snug sports bras and other fashionable yet tight pushups will send a signal to the brain to slow milk production and can also cause plugged ducts and breast infections.

- Unless you have very large or heavy breasts, underwires are unnecessary and best avoided. They can restrict milk production and flow. If you must purchase one, select a bra that fits properly and allows for room behind and beyond the milk ducts that extend past your armpits.

- Choose a breathable cotton bra without moisture-resistant liners. Trapped moisture can breed yeast or bacterial growth. If you will be using nursing pads, it isn't necessary to have one built into your bra.

- Purchase a bra with several rows of hooks, or buy a bra extension to wear during the first two weeks. These are the straps of fabric that are lined with additional hooks that fasten to the back of your bra. They can turn a 36 band-size bra into a 40. Your breasts will change again once your routine is established, but for now you'll need a tool to support your expanding bustline.

When you find a bra that meets all of your criteria, buy two or three of the same kind. You'll be washing them frequently, so you'll want one available at any given time.

Pads

Nursing pads are a godsend for mothers with a fast milk ejection reflex. You may be standing in line at the grocery store when something triggers your letdown. Maybe it's the sound or smell of an infant. Maybe it's a picture of a baby. Your breasts may achieve letdown like squirt guns. Nursing pads are your protective barrier against public embarrassment. The most cost-effective pads are made of cotton or terry cloth and can be laundered and reused. Some are formfitting to give you extra shapeliness.

Cutting a disposable diaper into sections to use as nursing pads will release moisture beads that expand with wetness. These are difficult to remove from your breast and are easily ingested by your baby. Although the beads are not poisonous, they aren't meant for human consumption!

All department stores sell nursing pads. They also market disposable pads with moisture-resistant plastic liners. When moisture gets trapped in the liners, bacteria and fungi can flourish in the warm, damp darkness. Who wants a petri dish in her bra? If you're on a budget, you can use cotton hankies or cut a cloth diaper to fit. Nursing pads just might give "stuffing your bra" a whole new meaning.

Pillows

You will use nursing pillows to help elevate your baby to your breast. You'll also use them to support your arms and back. (Some mothers love the Boppy pillow.) Most nursing pillows will continue to be useful as your baby grows. At about five to six months, your baby can use your pillow for supported sitting.

Slings or Blankets

Slings are a must for discreet nursing in public, and they offer a convenient way to tote baby around the house. Most slings are made of a three-foot-long piece of cotton fabric that you can adjust to "wear" your baby in several positions as he grows. (Most will hold up to about thirty-five pounds.) Traditionally, slings are used in countries where women continue to work with their baby attached at the hip. In the United States, slings are a relatively new idea, but they've become the fashion choice for veteran breastfeeders.

FIGURE 4-4:
Sling

Like baby hammocks, slings support your baby's spine and keep it aligned. Research has shown that babies carried by sling, kept close to their parents, cry less, are more calm, have stronger attachment formation, and are more in sync with Mom's movements.

You can wear double slings if you have twins. Think of them as baby bandoleers. The best part about slings is that you can walk around nursing your baby, and no one will know. You may opt for blankets instead, and those are just as handy. They can easily be used to shelter a nursing baby and double as warmers in a cold car seat.

Pumps

If you plan to return to work, or just want a reliable breast pump, make your purchase now. There are many different types and brands. You will need to choose a model that's both efficient and cost-effective. Renting is another option. Call your hospital lactation consultant, WIC office, or local breast pump depot for information. The best breast pumps are pretty pricey, but they are a good investment if you intend to use them. Some women have purchased cheap, battery-operated handheld pumps that destroy breast tissue, while others have invested in professional- or hospital-grade pumps that grew cobwebs in the closet. Again, have a good idea of what your needs are, and choose the best pump for your circumstances.

Footstool

Babies need a lap to nurse. Create a comfortable lap by using a footstool. They eliminate stress on your legs, back, and shoulders. You can improvise by using any item that's sturdy enough to support your feet and legs. Try a coffee table, a pile of books, or a cardboard box. If you're discussing the purchase of a new rocking chair or glider, a matching footstool is worth the extra money.

Breast Shells

Breast shells won't be necessary for everyone, but if you have flat or inverted nipples, they will be an important purchase. They also help if you have sore or cracked nipples from improper latch. You can find these through your hospital lactation consultant or department store, or buy them at most online baby stores.

Burp Cloths

It's a time-honored truth: Babies are moist. Whether you breastfeed or bottle feed, your baby will spit up. A couple of dozen cloth diapers are a wise, inexpensive, and necessary investment. Cloth diapers are thick, absorbent, and cost less than a new wardrobe.

Nursing Fashions

Once your baby arrives, you'll move into the exciting world of nursing fashions! You'll want to purchase two-piece outfits that allow for easy breast access. You may choose blouses that button or those that can be lifted. Oversized tops, sweatshirts, leggings, capris, and spandex become the nursing mother's uniform. Comfort is vital. You'll want to avoid dry-clean only fabrics and replace them with washable, breathable cottons and other fabrics that don't trap moisture. Prints tend to hide the telltale bull's-eyes of breastmilk leakage that solids only emphasize.

Labor Medications and Breastfeeding

Discuss labor pain management with your midwife or doctor. Ask your doctor what she recommends. During labor, you need to be free to concentrate on the task at hand and not on making last-minute decisions.

Your choices for pain relief will be either pharmacological (drugs) or nonpharmacological (nondrugs). Ask your provider to explain the risks and the benefits of the various methods she employs as well as the effects they have on breastfeeding. A fast, relatively easy labor might require only support and encouragement. A long, difficult labor might require the use of many different options.

The most common types of pharmacological interventions include:

Morphine. Morphine is frequently used to help anxious mothers relax, or when prolonged labor is anticipated. It is administered by injection, in an IV, or in an epidural catheter. It makes Mom sleepy and crosses the placenta, making baby sleepy, too. There is often a decrease in fetal heart accelerations, and it usually slows the process of labor.

Demerol. Demerol can cause respiratory depression in both mother and baby, one of the leading causes for emergency caesarean sections. Demerol frequently causes nausea or vomiting. It also reduces available oxygen for the baby. More than any other drug used in labor, Demerol has been shown to delay initiation of breastfeeding, but that's only because someone conducted a study on Demerol and breastfeeding specifically.

Stadol and Nubain. These narcotics cause dizziness and sleepiness, after an initial buzz that sends you into space. Subsequent doses have little or no effect because your body gets used to Stadol quickly, so it just doesn't work the second time around. While these medications are less likely to cause breathing problems for the baby, their relief duration is short.

Epidural anesthesia. Epidural anesthesia consists of injections of small amounts of anesthetics near the spinal nerves. This method eliminates pain in some areas of your body but allows you to remain alert throughout the birth of your baby. Unfortunately, it also weakens your contractions and slows labor. You often don't feel the urge to push and the experience of giving birth is something you might feel you have missed.

FACTS

Labor medications will cross the placental wall and enter your baby's bloodstream. The effects of these medications can cause your infant to have a delayed latch or uncoordinated suckling. Your baby may have a hard time getting to the breast if he's sleepy from drugs. Combining medications seems to increase this effect, especially for the first twelve hours after delivery.

The most common types of nonpharmacological interventions are:

Pattern-paced breathing. This type of breathing is one of the relaxation techniques you learned in childbirth education class. Your mantra will start out as "hee hee hee ho" and end with "I want to go home NOW!"

Hot-and-cold therapy. The use of heated rice socks, blankets, and ice packs are natural ways to stop pain receptors from signaling the brain. They also provide competing sensations that decrease your awareness of pain.

Massage and accupressure. These techniques work in much the same way as hot-and-cold therapy. Accupressure stimulates a set of nerve impulses that interrupts pain signals. Massage relaxes and releases tension. Scented massage oils provide aromatherapy for the body and brain.

Changing positions. When you're medicated, you become a health risk and a hospital liability. That's why laboring women were traditionally confined to their hospital bed. Lying flat on your back throughout labor was not nature's plan. When you can walk or use a birthing ball, gravity assists you by expanding your pelvic cavity so your baby can descend more quickly and efficiently. Unrestricted movement decreases labor duration.

Water therapy. Hydrotherapy is a tool that relieves discomfort in labor. Water is relaxing in almost any form. It has proven effective in relieving high blood pressure and backache. Many women labor in the bathtub and give birth in special pools.

A large part of the decision you make about pain relief depends on your perspective and attitude about the birth process (is it a natural event or a medically managed condition?) and your confidence in your ability to labor and give birth. Recently, a group of midwives found that fewer than half of the women who started labor naturally needed pain medication. Unmedicated births make for more alert babies who are eager to initiate breastfeeding and have a stronger, more coordinated suck.

Breastfeeding and Your Birth Plan

Hospitals and birthing centers are now striving to become more maternal-friendly. They encourage patients to be partners in their own health care. One way to accomplish this goal is through the use of birth plans.

Birth plans are written statements that allow you to make informed decisions about labor, delivery, and newborn procedures before your baby arrives. They are based on both current information and available options. These plans open the door for communication with your doctor. There are interactive birth plans available on several Web sites.

It is important to remember that most plans are based on idealized births. Your birthing experience will almost certainly fall somewhere in the middle. You can plan for the best, but expect that there may be a revision or two, if medically necessary, and be flexible enough to allow for it.

The Nouns: People, Places, and Things

When formulating your birth plan, you'll have several factors to consider, from who will be attending the birth to where you hope to have it to what labor methods you will use. Discuss your options with your partner and your doctor to determine what works best for you.

THE PEOPLE

Who will attend your birth?

Are partners, siblings, and extended family welcome?

Will you use a doula?

Will residents and students be allowed to breeze in and out during the process?

Will your birth partner be present for all newborn care procedures?

THE PLACES

Will your labor take place at the hospital, birth center, or home?

Will you labor, give birth, and recover in the same room?

Does this room come equipped with a squat bar, birthing bed, or whirlpool?

Will baby room with you fully, partially, or not at all?

THE THINGS

Will you labor naturally or use medications?

What interventions are acceptable to you (induction, forceps, vacuum, internal fetal monitoring)?

What labor methods are approved and supported by your provider (birthing ball, full or restricted movement, hydrotherapy)?

Remember that a birthing plan is the starting point for you and your doctor. You'll be otherwise occupied during delivery, so it's important that the other people involved know your wishes and intentions.

Your Breastfeeding Plan

You will want to make a special note in your birth plan that you intend to breastfeed. It is important to have this in writing, but tell your doctor as well as the nursery staff. If you're using a doula, she will be the first to help your baby to the breast, and she will keep hospital staff informed.

You will want to include the following in your plan:

1. Please do not offer my baby formula, glucose (sugar water), pacifiers, or artificial nipples.
2. My primary feeding preference is exclusive breastfeeding.
3. I would like the assistance of a lactation consultant or breastfeeding

educator to help me establish a nursing routine before I leave the birthing facility.

4. In the event that my baby needs medical interventions, I would like to provide expressed breastmilk.

Some newborn-care nurses may recommend offering your baby a glucose or formula supplement. Have Dad advocate for you.

> Fathers are your greatest advocate! Dad can make sure your baby isn't given pacifiers, formula, or glucose, and he can stand up against hospital policies that aren't breastfeeding-friendly.

Sugar water and formula will fill baby's tummy so he won't be hungry when you offer your breast for feeding. Babies given supplements aren't learning how to breastfeed. They are learning how to feed from a bottle. However, there are situations that might require supplementation with formula for medical emergencies (see Chapter 10). If your baby is unable to nurse, your lactation consultant will work with you to express colostrum for use.

The use of pacifiers should also be identified in your birth plan. Pacifiers will satisfy your baby's sucking reflex, but you need your baby's suckle to help develop your milk supply. Pacifiers will only hinder this process. Pacifiers should not be introduced until at least six weeks after birth or until a solid nursing routine has been established.

The Use of Doulas

Many couples are now employing the services of qualified doulas to assist them with labor, birth, and postpartum care. A prenatal doula is a professional labor assistant who:

- Acts as a liaison between medical staff and the laboring couple.
- Views childbirth as a natural event and not a medically managed condition.

- Guides your birth partner in providing natural relief, support, and encouragement to you during labor.
- Helps you develop your birth plan and advocates for its use.
- Provides comfort measures.
- Records all aspects of your birth story.

Doulas are very much like nurturing Earth Mothers. Both moms and dads report more favorable birth experiences with the use of a qualified labor assistant. Dads often find the experience much more positive and pleasurable and far less stress inducing when another person is present to share the task of providing comfort and support.

Both prenatal and postpartum doulas are available to help you establish a breastfeeding routine. Your prenatal doula won't leave your side until your baby is placed at your breast and latched on properly. Your postpartum doula will assist with newborn care, breastfeeding, emotional support, and, sometimes, light household assistance. They provide home-based services because home is the environment where you will raise your baby.

FACTS

Studies on the use of doulas have found a 50 percent reduction in Caesarean rates, 25 percent decrease in labor duration, 60 percent reduction in epidural use, 40 percent reduction in oxytocin induction, 30 percent decrease in the need for labor medications, 40 percent reduction in forceps deliveries, as well as fewer birth complications, lower rates of postpartum depression, increased breastfeeding success, more positive newborn assessments, and greater reported satisfaction with the childbirth experience.

Most doulas charge between $200 and $800 per delivery and accept payment on a sliding fee scale or through a payment plan. Currently, Doulas of North America (DONA) is working on insurance reimbursement for families who use this service. You can find a certified doula by contacting DONA, your childbirth educator, or your doctor.

Breastfeeding Classes

Another very helpful option in preparation for breastfeeding is to attend a breastfeeding class. They are offered at your local hospital, through private maternal health organizations, or through your local WIC office. WIC not only offers classes for low- and middle-income families, but it can also refer you to local resources that support breastfeeding.

Most hospitals offer breastfeeding classes free of charge once or twice per week. Some classes are offered for pregnant couples who want more information about the techniques involved in nursing infants, while other classes focus on common concerns you have with your newborn. You might attend both. Postpartum breastfeeding classes offer one-on-one support with lactation consultants who answer questions and demonstrate new techniques.

Choosing a Pediatrician

Locate a pediatrician who supports breastfeeding. Almost all do, but some are too quick to offer formula or weaning as solutions when other options are available. The AAP has published its philosophy about the benefits of breastfeeding, encouraging mothers to nurse for six months exclusively and for as long as they want to after that.

It's important to find a pediatrician who has a wide knowledge base about breast anatomy, as well as personal experience with breastfeeding in general. Ask your provider why he supports breastfeeding, whom he refers to for potential problems, when he recommends weaning, and how many breastfeeding families are involved with his practice. Your provider will develop a health history with your child over the next several years. You can afford to be picky about whom you will partner with.

CHAPTER 5

Breastfeeding Basics

Immediately after birth and barring any complications, your doctor or midwife will lay your newborn on your tummy and you'll greet each other for the very first time. Your baby will be alert and the sound of your voice will captivate her. She will turn her head to listen to her mommy and daddy, and your voices will calm her cries within seconds. She might even try to vocalize in response to your soothing coos.

The First Hour

If breastfeeding is in your birth plan, your nurse or midwife will immediately place your baby at your breast to help involute your uterus and expel your placenta (or afterbirth). Nipple stimulation from your baby's suckling will cause your uterus to contract, which will gently squeeze the placenta to separate it from the uterine wall. It takes usually two to five contractions to deliver the placenta. Oxytocin is produced naturally when your baby nurses; it helps the uterus to contract, which controls blood loss and the risk of hemorrhage.

FACTS

Newborns are hardwired for breastfeeding. They can zero in on the darkened bull's-eye of the areola and can see your face clearly while nursing at your breast. Babies nuzzle the nipple aggressively to make it erect for latching on. They also have the ability to "crawl" to the breast within the first hour after birth and to memorize the smell of your breastmilk.

While your care provider is busy delivering the placenta, clamping and cutting the umbilical cord, repairing any tears to the perineum, and completing documentation, you and your baby will be exploring each other through rich sensory contact. You'll be counting her fingers and toes, and she'll be committing your scent to memory. Studies have shown that babies can identify their mothers from just the smell of their milk. Your baby is also satisfying her sucking reflex. This is the beginning of a beautiful relationship that will last a lifetime.

At the Hospital

In your birth plan, you noted that you intended to breastfeed. If you haven't already, now is the time to meet with a lactation consultant. A lactation consultant is a professional in the art of breastfeeding. Lactation consultants take international board exams to become licensed to practice, just as lawyers take the bar exam to practice law. They're recognized as top-level professionals in their field.

Most hospitals have a lactation consultant on staff, but in smaller or rural facilities, postpartum care nurses or certified breastfeeding educators will assist you if a lactation consultant is unavailable. These talented and caring people are there to instruct you in every aspect of breastfeeding, from positioning to latch to assessment. They'll show you how to nurse your baby and will provide support because they want you to succeed! If you happen to have a video camera handy, tape their demonstrations. They'll be invaluable when you go home and are on your own.

Ask

Ask questions. No question is too silly, stupid, or small. If the answer is vague or you just don't understand, ask your lactation consultant to slow down and speak in real-world terms. Don't hesitate to seek clarification. Have Dad, your labor coach, or another support person take notes for you or take this book with you and jot notes in the margins.

ESSENTIALS

If you are unclear about anything, ask again. Don't be intimidated by a busy hospital or a buzzing nurse. This is your time. What you learn now can determine your immediate breastfeeding success.

Watch

Observe and pay close attention as your lactation consultant or nurse demonstrates positions and steps involved in putting your baby to your breast. You'll have the opportunity to practice nursing several times before you leave the hospital. The repetition will be useful. Reading about a technique and watching it in action are two completely different things.

Listen

Your lactation consultant will share vital information with you. Stop what you're doing, make eye contact, and actively listen to what she has to say. Draw pictures in your mind as she explains the process.

Practice

Practice, then practice again. We retain 90 percent of what we're learning when we can demonstrate it and talk about it at the same time. Go through each step and describe what you are doing and why it is important.

Hospital staff will bring the baby to you for feeding every two to three hours around the clock. If your baby is rooming in with you, the hospital staff will remind you to nurse often. This will increase your milk supply and will also help you retain what you've learned about breastfeeding.

Before you leave the medical facility, inquire about hospital-grade breast pump rentals. Ask your lactation consultant to recommend a model and to demonstrate its use. If you return to work and want to express your milk, or have a special needs baby and need to pump, you'll want a high-quality breast pump for home and/or business use. Pumps come in all makes and models (see Chapter 12.) Your lactation consultant can show you the best pumps to purchase or rent.

At Home

When you first arrive home with your new baby, you might feel a little nervous or awkward about breastfeeding on your own. "Test anxiety" is perfectly normal when you're doing it for the first time on your own.

First and foremost, relax! Feel confident in your ability to do this! Keep this book close by for reference and feel free to contact your postpartum care nurse or lactation consultant for a final run through. The first couple of weeks take practice, but by the time you go in for your postpartum checkup, you'll have nursing down to an art.

When to Feed

You'll receive a lot of advice (wanted or not) about how to feed your baby over the next couple of months. You'll be asked if you are feeding "on schedule" or "on demand." On demand is a term used to describe your baby's biological cycle. On schedule usually means by the clock. In the first few days after birth, you will be doing both.

Frequency

How often you feed will be determined by your baby. If she is allowed to follow her own body rhythms throughout her life, she is less likely to be an overweight adult. Feeding on demand will also establish a strong milk supply. Babies know when they are hungry. They will demonstrate hunger cues when they are ready to eat. Put simply, babies eat when they are hungry and they stop when they are full. The only clock your baby cares about is her own body clock.

ALERT

If, after a week, your baby is still sleepy, take her to your doctor or midwife for a jaundice assessment. If she has yellow skin, yellow in the whites of her eyes, brick-red or dark urine, pale stools, or feeds poorly, she might need bilirubin lights, a form of photo therapy.

At the same time, babies in their first week of life are very sleepy, particularly if labor medications were used during the birth process. If your baby isn't waking on her own every two to three hours during the first week, you'll need to wake her to breastfeed. Now you're feeding on schedule or "by the clock."

After the first week of life, your baby will be more wakeful and will begin to tune into her own body rhythms. Until then, you will have to rouse her to reinforce the feeding pattern.

Schedule

During the early days, you'll realize that there is no schedule. Your baby has her own internal gas gauge. Her body will tell her when she's hungry and she'll show you by demonstrating hunger cues. Your baby is ready to eat when she exhibits these behaviors:

- Brings her clenched fist to her mouth
- Begins sucking on her fist or fingers
- Roots by turning her head to find your nipple
- Displays increased activity or movement
- Vocalizes and begins to make noise

Crying is a late hunger cue. If you wait until babies cry, you've waited too long. Identifying early hunger cues is an important part of learning to "read" your baby's behavior. Knowledge is power. Anticipate that she will be hungry when she wakes up, or when she displays these cues.

How Long to Feed

Offer one breast first, and when baby is finished, offer the second. Women were once advised to let their babies nurse for just ten minutes at each breast. Recent research suggests that the Ten Minute Rule no longer applies. The composition of breastmilk changes during a single feeding session and your baby needs both the foremilk and the hindmilk you produce. The foremilk comes quickly and is higher in volume and protein and lower in fat. The hindmilk is higher in fat and calories, but there's less of it. It's like having steak and ice cream, dinner and dessert. Babies need both.

Alternate the starting lineup at each feeding. Your baby might prefer one breast to the other, and that's normal. It might have to do with the position you hold her, the flow of milk, or any number of factors. You might prefer one breast to the other for the same reasons. However, it is essential to alternate your breasts to ensure a good milk supply.

Feed for as long as your baby is interested, fifteen to thirty minutes on average. If your baby is a marathon nurser on one breast, it could indicate that she is not latched on properly or there's a problem with your milk supply. However, babies approach nursing differently. It's a lot like eating ice cream . . . some of us lick and savor, while others bite and swallow. It rarely takes more than a maximum of twenty minutes per breast to "empty" it. Some babies will continue to nurse for comfort.

Most experts will tell you to feed your infant for fifteen minutes on each breast, but watch your baby and not the clock. It's more important for your baby to remove your milk than it is to follow a predetermined time limit.

Breastmilk is very digestible, so breastfed babies eat more often than formula-fed babies. In the first weeks, your baby will eat smaller amounts, but frequently. Later on, your baby will eat more and will reduce the number of feedings. Growth spurts happen around three weeks, six weeks, three months, and six months, and usually last about seven to ten days. During this time, you might notice that your baby eats more, and more frequently. Frequent feedings not only satisfy your baby, but they tell your body to make more milk in preparation for your baby's growing demands.

Baby at Your Breast: The Basics

Are you ready to begin? Eventually, both you and your baby will be old pros. Until you've mastered your technique, however, follow these simple steps for successful breastfeeding. With practice and patience, you'll be nursing like a pro in no time!

Getting Ready

It's important to remember to wash your hands just before nursing. The Montgomery glands will keep your nipples clean, but it's essential to practice good hygiene when handling both your breasts and your newborn.

Don't forget your water! There's something about nursing that makes women thirsty, so have a beverage available. Water is the best choice, but juice or decaffeinated teas are healthy, too. Avoid caffeine, as it can reduce your milk supply and cause tummy upset for your baby.

Find a comfortable place that will become your nursing nest: a couch, a rocker, or your bed. Use pillows to support your elbows, arms, and back. Use a footrest, a telephone book, or last week's laundry to support your feet. Rocking chairs with footrests are perfect, but feel free to improvise with what you have available. It's important that you're comfortable. You may be there for a while.

Get Your Costar

Bring your baby close to you, chest to breast, using the position that works best for both of you. Your baby's body will face you. Use pillows to bring her up to the level of your breast. Nursing pillows, bed pillows, rolled blankets, baby slings, or couch cushions will offer your baby support and the height she needs. It's important that when you are chest to breast with your baby, her ear, shoulder, and hip form a straight line. Turn your head and try to swallow. It's not easy and it's uncomfortable! That's why it's important to have your baby's body aligned (ear, shoulder, hip).

Bring your baby to the breast, not the breast to your baby. Don't lean forward to offer your breast. Instead, with one hand cradling her head, your forearm supporting her back and hips, and the other hand holding your breast, pull your baby to you.

Support your breast with a C hold, like the way you hold a hamburger, only upside down. When we eat, we use our hands to shape and contour the sandwich. The same principles apply here. Support your breast with your thumb on top positioned behind the areola and the weight of your breast in your hand. After a while, you might not need to continue this hold throughout the entire feeding, but if you have large or heavy breasts, they'll benefit from the support. If your hand seems awkward, place a rolled up towel under your breast for support.

The All-Important Latch

Encourage her to open her mouth as wide as possible, as if she were yawning. You might tickle her cheek or bottom lip to stimulate her rooting reflex, if needed. In one sweeping motion, pull baby toward you to position her at your breast. Center your nipple over your baby's tongue, aim your nipple toward the roof of her mouth, and bring her chin to your breast.

Latching on correctly is the most critical key to breastfeeding success. This part takes some practice. Your baby should take the entire nipple and most of the areola into her mouth. If you have large areolas, make sure she's getting about one inch of it into her mouth. More areola should be visible at the top of your breast than at the bottom. Latching on is not symmetrical. Note where her lower lip makes contact. It's the lower jaw that actually extracts the milk as she compresses the milk sinuses. Your nipple should be centered over her tongue. If it just doesn't feel right or it hurts, pull baby's lower lip back enough to see if her tongue is properly positioned over her lower gum line. If you can't see it, or if you hear a clicking noise when she nurses, she might be sucking her tongue in addition to your breast. Break the latch and reposition.

Your baby will take your nipple to the back of her throat. As she works her bottom jaw to compress the milk sinuses, milk trickles down the back of her throat. It's similar to the way you would suck your thumb.

FIGURE 5-1: A proper latch

FIGURE 5-2: Breaking the latch

Breaking the Latch

Break the latch by inserting your finger into your baby's mouth at the inside cheek to release suction. Hook the nipple and draw it out as you pull your breast away. Baby might try to relatch, but if your hooked finger is covering your nipple, she can't. If you allow your baby to slide off the nipple while she's still creating suction, you'll have sore or cracked nipples. Breaking the latch will be a smooth process once you have tried it a couple of times.

LATCH EVALUATION CHECKLIST

❑ Does your baby have the entire nipple and at least one inch of the areola in her mouth?

❑ After your milk lets down, can you hear your baby swallow?

❑ Does baby follow a "suck, suck, suck, swallow" pattern?

❑ Do you hear a clicking sound that indicates improper latch?

❑ Can you see noticeable movement in her jaw all the way to her ear (ear wiggling)?

❑ Is the area at her temple moving?

❑ Are her lips flanged or everted around the nipple?

If you feel pain (excluding the tingling sensation of letdown), break the latch and reposition. If your baby is taking in only the nipple, break the latch and reposition. If something just doesn't feel right, break the latch and reposition.

Breastfeeding should not be painful. If your baby is positioned on your areola correctly, you should not feel anything more than a slight tug. Pain is often the result of nipple feeding, and continued nipple feeding will lead to cracked or sore nipples and even greater discomfort.

Suck, Suck, Suck, Swallow

Babies breastfeed in rhythm. At first they suck steadily and somewhat aggressively to stimulate your milk ejection reflex. As the jaw moves up and down against the breast sinuses to extract milk, you'll begin to notice a pattern to your baby's nursing. She might suck from four to ten times, pause for about five or ten seconds, then continue this pattern for about three to five minutes. This pattern stimulates the letdown of your hindmilk. Once this happens, you will be able to hear her swallow. Her rhythm changes to suck, suck, suck, swallow, pause, suck, suck, suck, swallow, pause. Once breastfeeding is established, letdown happens more quickly.

The flow of a fast milk ejection reflex can sometimes be more than your baby can handle. You might notice milk dripping from her mouth or she might cough and need to catch her breath. If she's sputtering, break the latch and take her off the breast just long enough for her to swallow, then begin again. After a few minutes you'll notice that her suck will begin to slow and she'll have longer pauses between sucks.

As babies tire and begin to nod off, there will be several very long pauses. But the minute you try to take your baby off the breast or stimulate her cheek, she'll almost always start to suck again. Often, by this time, baby has slid off the areola and is nipple feeding, not breastfeeding. Break the latch and start again.

Labor Again?

Early on, you will feel uterine contractions when your baby begins to nurse. These are called afterpains. You might feel a gush of blood on your sanitary pad at the same time. With nipple stimulation, your uterus regains its tone and dispels excess blood. These same contractions also shrink your uterus to its prepregnant pear size.

If this is your second or third baby, your contractions might feel stronger than before. Practice the breathing patterns you used in childbirth education classes. After a few weeks, these contractions will cease.

Ending a Feeding

When your baby is done with the first breast, burp her, change her diaper if necessary, then offer her the second breast. However, she might fall asleep without finishing the second breast. It will be important to remember to start on the unfinished side the next time your baby nurses.

Breastfeeding Positions

After your baby arrives, both of you will find a technique that works for you. You'll also discover your preference for positions after some practice.

It is important that you feel comfortable with at least one of the positions listed below. Here are a few different options for you to try.

Cradle Position

The cradle position is the most commonly used position during the first few weeks of life. Because we tend to be cautious about holding our newborns, we tend to choose positions that allow us more control. In the cradle position, as in all breastfeeding positions, the baby's ear, shoulder, and hip will form a line and baby will be chest to breast with you. Chest to breast means that you turn your baby toward you so her chest is even with your breast (and sometimes her foot will be in your armpit if she's especially active). Use pillows to cushion your baby in your lap. Baby needs to have her head and mouth at the same height as your nipple.

Your baby's head will be on your forearm (at the crook of your elbow) and her back will be along your inner arm. The palm of your hand will support her bottom. If you are preparing to breastfeed on the left breast, your right hand supports the breast in a C hold. You support your baby with your left arm and hand. Pull your baby to the breast with your forearm. Use pillows to cushion your elbows.

FIGURE 5-3:
Cradle hold

FIGURE 5-4:
Cross-cradle position

Cross-Cradle Position

This is another excellent method and the one used most frequently while learning the art of breastfeeding. The cross-cradle gives you maximum control in holding your baby and bringing her to the breast. If nursing on the right side, gently place your left hand behind your baby's ears with your thumb and index finger, behind each ear. Your baby's neck rests in the web between the thumb, index finger, and palm of your hand. The palm of your hand is positioned between her shoulder blades. Your right hand supports your breast in the C position.

Again, use pillows to support baby and your arms. As you begin the latch, be sure baby's mouth is close to your nipple and at the same height. When baby opens her mouth, bring her to your nipple with the palm of your hand from between her shoulder blades.

Football Hold

This is a great position for a mother who has had a Caesarean birth, has large breasts, or has a very large or premature baby. Most newborns are comfortable in this position, too. To use the football hold, place baby on her side at your side. You will support your baby's head in your hand and her back along your arm as you did in the cross-cradle hold, but this time the baby is beside you and her legs are tucked under your arm. Continue to support your breast with a C hold using the opposite hand.

FIGURE 5-5: Football hold

FIGURE 5-6: Side-lying position

Side-Lying Position

Many moms use the side-lying position to nurse their babies at night or if they are on bedrest for medical reasons. In this position, you can bring baby to bed with you and nurse while lying down. Both you and your baby lie on your sides facing each other, chest to breast. Baby is cradled in your arm with her head in the crook of your elbow. Her back is supported by the forearm on the same side you're nursing on. Baby's hip, shoulder, and ear form a line. Use pillows to support your head, back, and legs during this feeding. If you are anxious about trying this position at night, practice during the day until you feel more comfortable. Roll a towel or blanket to place behind your baby to support her back.

Over the Shoulder

If you have extremely large or heavy breasts, this position is the one that sometimes saves the breastfeeding relationship. Lie flat on your back on the floor or the bed. Position your baby over your shoulder so that she's lying tummy to shoulder with you. She is positioned facedown over the nipple. You can monitor the latch from your position in the nosebleed section up above. If you have very large breasts and doubt your ability to perform these gymnastic feats, talk to a lactation consultant. She will guide you through the proper positioning to make breastfeeding successful.

ESSENTIALS   If you are still pregnant and have a doll available, practice holding positions and the art of bringing baby to breast.

Using a variety of positions helps to work the breast from all angles and empties the breast more efficiently, reducing the risk of plugged ducts. With time, you and your baby will find a feeding pattern that works best. Perhaps you're right-handed and have found the cross-cradle position on the left breast most comfortable and the football hold on the right breast the best position.

Burping

Breastfed babies usually take in less air with their feedings than bottle-fed infants. But all babies need to be burped or they will cry when air bubbles sit in their tummies. Here are a few of the most common methods of burping a baby.

Over-the-shoulder burping. Hold baby against your chest with her head over your shoulder. Gently rub or pat her back until she burps.

Sitting-upright burping. Sit baby on your knee and support her with the spread fingers of your hand on her chest. Use the web area of your hand to support her chin. The other hand supports her back as you gently pat her back to burp her.

Over-the-lap burping. Place baby on her tummy and across your lap. Pat or rub her back until she burps. Take care not to bounce your legs as this will upset her tummy and she'll spit up on your shoes.

FIGURE 5-7:
Over the shoulder

FIGURE 5-8:
Sitting upright

FIGURE 5-9:
Over the lap

Burping should be slow and relatively gentle. You'll find that light patting and rubbing should produce the desired results within a few minutes. As with all the rest of the breastfeeding and burping routines, you will learn to understand what's "normal" for your baby over time.

Spitup

Although breastfed babies spit up less often than formula-fed infants, you can still expect to have a little of your breastmilk returned to you. Don't be alarmed if your baby occasionally spews. It may look like she spit up her entire meal, but it's often not as much as it appears. Take a tablespoon of water and dump it on the counter. It might look like a lot, but considering your baby is taking in two or more ounces at a single feeding, a tablespoon is a drop in the bucket. However, any projectile vomiting should be reported to your doctor.

CHAPTER 6
Fine-Tuning

Just when you think you know so much, there are so many more things to consider. Breastfeeding is not just mealtime for your baby—it requires comfort, quiet, and relaxation for both of you. Your location, routine, and attitude all play a part in a positive and successful experience. Don't forget that over time, breastfeeding will become less complicated as you and your baby find your groove.

Your Breastfeeding Environment

Comfort is key for your breastfeeding environment. You'll want to set up a special place for your "nursing nest." Whether it's a favorite rocking chair in a corner of your living room, a space in the baby's nursery, or even your bed, a relaxed and calm atmosphere makes the best nursing nest. The following are some ideas to consider when choosing your place:

Burping cloths—Keep your supply of burping cloths close by. You might use several at each feeding in the first few weeks, so have at least a dozen or so within easy reach of your chair or bed.

Chair—Whether it's a stuffed recliner, a decorative glider, or a wooden rocker, your chair should be comfortable. You'll need support for your back and arms as well as your legs. You'll be using the chair for long periods of time throughout the day and night, so look for one that you like.

Climate—Your home should be kept at a temperature that's comfortable for everyone. Your nursing nest should be strategically placed away from drafts in the winter and hot or stuffy spots in the summer. Pay attention to the location of heating and cooling vents or radiators. The temperature near heating and cooling outlets varies a lot more than it does elsewhere in the room. Finally, keep a blanket handy for both of you.

Drink—Take one with you and keep it within easy reach. It's inevitable that you'll become thirsty when your baby starts to nurse.

Lighting—Try to pick a location that allows you to control the lighting. You'll want to keep the room dimly lit at night and at nap times. Bright lights don't seem to bother nursing babies, but they might make it more difficult for you to relax. A table lamp near your chair or bed is perfect. Windows should be curtained or shaded, both for light control and privacy. Avoid windows that face east. When the morning sun shines through the east windows at 6:00 A.M., you and your baby might find it more difficult to go back to bed for that last stolen hour of sleep.

Magazine—Reading a magazine or a book while your baby nurses is a pleasant way to pass the time. You can keep up on world events, read about the joys of parenting, or just get lost for a while in a good novel. Breastfeeding gives you plenty of quiet, guilt-free reading time.

Music/TV—Listening to music or watching your favorite shows can help you relax.

Pillows—You'll need pillows for support as well as to raise your lap.

Table—You'll need a table to hold your drink, remote control, book, and perhaps a breast pump. A sturdy end table or a coffee table will work. You might want to have a phone handy, as well as the phone numbers of your health care providers.

Like sitting down to do anything, getting settled to breastfeed will require a bit of planning and a bit of compromise. You'll forget the phone. Or the remote control. Or the nursing pillow. You'll know soon enough which accessories you can live without—and which are critical to success.

Establishing a Routine

Newborn routine is an oxymoron. As days melt into nights and you're walking in a twilight slumber, you'll wish your newborn knew what routine meant. But with the passing weeks, things will change and your baby will develop a fairly predictable schedule for eating, sleeping, playing, and eliminating. You'll become more in tune with your infant's cues and able to anticipate what will follow next.

There is value in routines. They give adults some sense of control, and as children get older, routines promote good habits and give kids a feeling of security and structure.

The Early Days

You might be waking your baby every two to three hours to feed, particularly in the first two weeks. You'll offer your baby your breast eight to twelve times in every twenty-four-hour period. Demand feeding won't begin until after your sleepy baby has had time to regulate her internal body clock, about two to three weeks after birth. At that time, you'll breastfeed as often as your baby wants. It might be anywhere between one and four hours, or it might be a series of evening cluster feeds. Your baby will let you know when she's hungry. However, during those early sleepy days, you'll be waking her to ensure that she has plenty of opportunities to eat, drink, and be merry.

QUESTIONS?

Should I provide formula supplements during my baby's growth spurts?
Supplemental feedings of formula are unnecessary. Cluster feedings can be unnerving, but they are a natural way for your baby to stimulate increased milk production, and for your breasts to meet that demand for your growing infant.

Around three weeks of age, some babies want to nurse every hour, particularly if they are entering a growth spurt. These frequent nursings are called cluster or bunch feeds. Babies seem to space their feedings closer together at certain times of the day or night, then wait long periods between nursing sessions. It seems that just as you're ready to take your baby from the breast, she begins to root again. Cluster feeds are usually followed by longer periods of uninterrupted deep sleep, a sign that your baby is going through a growth spurt. Cluster feedings can cause a new mother to wonder if she's producing enough milk for her hungry baby. They can also try a mom's patience, but the phase is usually temporary (until the next time).

This is the way you will be developing your newborn "routine" for the next couple of weeks:

You will watch your baby.	>	Your baby will give hunger cues.
You will position your baby, chest to chest.	>	Your baby takes position to nurse.
You prepare to latch baby to your breast.	>	Your baby latches on.
You drink according to thirst.	>	Your baby nurses to satiety.
You feel sleepy.	>	Your baby feels sleepy, too!

When your baby begins to doze or flutter suck after feeding for some time, burp her and offer her the second breast. Your baby will probably have a bowel movement once or twice during the nursing session. The diaper change can correspond with the breast switch.

Moving On

It might take up to three weeks before you learn to read your infant's cues well, but you will. Soon, you'll be a pro at interpreting even her most subtle of cues, as only a parent can.

As your baby gets older, you'll begin to establish other routines as well. Your bedtime routine may include activities like a bath, a massage, a story, soft music or lullabies, rocking, and a bedtime snack. Start bedtime routines early in life so your baby will begin to make associations between these transitions and sleep. But choose your bedtime routine carefully. You might not mind an hour-long process now, but in a few years, it might lose some of its charm. Many of the bedtime routines you establish now will become steadfast habits when your baby grows into a toddler.

Your Baby's Sleep/Wake Cycle

Babies don't know if it's day or night. They tell time, not by a clock or sundial, but by their own internal regulators. Infants move through predictable states of arousal every day. This is called the sleep/wake cycle, and it includes six states that your baby will move through in sequence.

State one. Quiet or deep sleep is characterized by little or no activity. You'll observe your baby's chest rising and falling rhythmically, a sign of deep relaxation. Your baby's eyelids will be closed, and she'll move very little. Babies in this state don't seem to have any awareness of light or sound. Every thirty to forty-five minutes, she might cycle between deep sleep and active sleep. When people say they sleep like a baby, this is what they mean!

State two. Active or light sleep is another sleep state. You'll see your baby's eyes darting around under her lids. This is called rapid eye movement (REM). You'll also notice her muscles twitching and facial expressions like smiling or frowning. Babies often make chewing motions or sucking sounds in light sleep.

State three. Drowsiness is a transitional state between sleep and waking. Babies have that dazed, unfocused, dreamy-eyed appearance while drowsy. Your baby's eyes might open and close, her breathing pattern is irregular, she might wake if stimulated, and might exhibit a startle response to loud noises.

State four. The quiet alert state is the best time to breastfeed or perform infant massage. Babies are relaxed, alert, focused, and observant, and they maintain good eye contact and have that "lover's gaze." Your baby is awake and ready for breakfast!

Even though your baby is small, it's important to change her positions and environment often throughout the day. Rocking, singing, talking, taking walks, massaging, playing on the floor, and being carried by sling all help to offer opportunities for your baby to explore! Intelligence is built like a pyramid. The broader the base, the higher the peak.

State five. Active alert is the state where your baby is busy. She begins to vocalize or "talk," she may become fussy, and her feet are constantly moving. She is easily overstimulated in this state, which can move her into the next: crying.

State six. Crying is a state, too. You'll know this one well after the first week. And after a while, you'll be able to distinguish between baby's cries of hunger, boredom, fatigue, pain, loneliness, and overstimulation. Sometimes, babies just need to blow off steam. Then they cycle back around to sleep.

Some babies transition smoothly from one state to the next, while others change so quickly you wonder if they have a diagnosable personality disorder. Your baby's transitioning style is, in part, due to personality and temperament.

In their first two weeks of life, babies eat and sleep, eat and sleep, eat and sleep. In their first week, they sleep an average of twelve to twenty hours per day.

SLEEP CHART			
	DAY	NIGHT	TOTAL
First Week	8–10	8–10	16–20
One Month	7–10	7–8	14–18
Three Months	6–8	6–8	12–16
Six Months	4–6	6–8	10–14
Nine Months	3–5	8–10	11–15
Twelve Months	2–4	8–10	10–14

This sleep schedule indicates hours of sleep in a twenty-four-hour period, not consecutive hours of sleep! If you manage to get four uninterrupted hours of sleep, count yourself lucky. Baby-care shifts work well during the early weeks, so both you and your partner have an opportunity to sleep undisturbed for a short period of time. Night sleep patterns do not mean after midnight, either. "Night" is anytime after the sun goes down. Sleep time will increase at night as your baby begins to eliminate naps.

Waking Your Sleepy Baby

Because babies spend their first two weeks in a sleepy state, they must be awakened every two to three hours for feeding. Frequent feedings mean a more abundant milk supply for you and healthy weight gain for your baby.

Here is a bag of tricks to wake your sleepy baby for feeding:

- Change her diaper or gently wipe her face or back with a cool washcloth.
- Gently stroke her mouth, cheeks, and lips.

- Hold her skin-to-skin with you or Dad.
- Hold her upright, under her arms, and, while supporting her neck and head, gently bounce her, sing to her, or offer her your clean finger to stimulate her sucking response.
- Lay her on her back and stimulate her skin with massage.
- Rub the palms of her hands and the soles of her feet.
- Try scalp massage by drawing small circles on her head with your fingers.
- Unswaddle your baby or remove her clothing.

You don't have to rouse her completely to a wide-awake state to nurse her, especially in the middle of the night. Keep the lights low and block out external noises that might startle her. She needs to be alert enough to nurse but not so much so that she has a hard time falling back to sleep.

Middle-of-the-Night Feedings

Perhaps the biggest adjustment new parents must make is their sleep schedule. Before your baby was born, you slept when you were tired and stayed in bed as long as you wanted. Now, the amount of sleep you get will depend on your baby.

Check your baby's sleeping environment for safety. Always place her on her back on a firm mattress. Don't use overstuffed blankets or comforters. Remove pillows and toys from your baby's crib. Keep the room temperature comfortable, neither hot nor cold. Dress baby for sleeping the same as you would dress yourself.

Your newborn doesn't have a set schedule, and even after he does, you'll be up several times in the night to feed him. The quality of your sleep will change. You'll sleep more lightly, almost with one eye open and one ear to the baby monitor. If you are cobedding, every little stir will rouse you.

You'll even develop a strategy with your spouse called the "I'm Sleeping, It's Your Turn" game. Here's how to play: Your baby calls out, but both parents lie quietly, pretending to be asleep. The first one who moves, loses. Your internal dialogue goes something like this, "Please, please get up. Can't you see I'm exhausted? I'm not moving. It's your turn. And if it's not your turn, it's still your turn! Get up!" Then, give your partner a subtle kick. Tag. "You're it."

If you're expressing milk, the diplomatic alternative is to simply trade nights or take shifts. You can work 10:00 P.M. to 2:00 A.M., and he gets 2:00 A.M. to 6:00 A.M.

ESSENTIALS

Instead of setting your alarm clock to wake you for midnight feedings, drink a full glass of water at bedtime. When you get up to go to the bathroom, pick up your baby for his night feeding. If you break into his sleep rhythm before he has a chance to fully wake up, you'll be able to get him back to sleep more easily.

Most babies wake two to three times to be fed throughout the night. Some sleep in four-hour stretches. (Those probably belong to the same moms who were never sick during pregnancy, had easy labors, and now look like they were never pregnant.) Keep external stimulation to a minimum, unless you're trying to wake a sleepy baby for a feeding.

Around six or seven months of age, or when solids are introduced, babies will often begin to sleep through the night. If they're offered a varied diet during the day, they might not need to feed at night as frequently as before. There's no hard and fast rule, though. Your baby will let you know when he needs to nurse.

The Family Bed

Cobedding has been a cultural practice for all but a few Western societies since the beginning of time. Japanese, Chinese, Indian, and other cultures shared beds with newborns as a way to give babies shelter and security. Even in the United States in times past, parents shared their beds with infants and toddlers. Suzanne's grandfather slept at the foot of his parents' bed, along with other siblings, until he was six years of age. It was a custom of the times, born out of need due to limited space, access to heat, and economics.

Popular Opinion

The idea of cobedding has received mixed reviews from health care providers, families, and society in general. It isn't for everyone, but it does have some tremendous benefits for breastfeeding families.

Breastfeeding mothers feel more in sync with their cobedding infants. They share the same sleep cycles, and mothers often report feeling more rested as a result. They approach nighttime feedings with a relaxed attitude, mind, and body. This ability to relax helps their milk ejection reflex work more effectively. Mothers simply gather their infants in their arms and side-lie as their babies nurse at the breast. Their babies often fall back asleep without completely entering an alert state.

Benefits for Baby

Studies have shown that babies who cobed cry less than babies who sleep alone. They also gain weight more consistently. In fact, one of the methods prescribed by doctors who diagnose breastfeeding problems is for Mom to simply take her infant to bed, to rest and nurse.

The family bed might even help reduce your baby's risk of sudden infant death syndrome (SIDS). Cobedding studies by Dr. James McKenna indicate that infants cobedding with their parents spend greater time in active or light sleep than infants who sleep alone. SIDS most often occurs when infants are in a state of deep sleep.

SSENTIALS

If you cobed with your baby, make sure your sleeping environment is as safe as her crib to prevent the risk of SIDS. Don't place babies on waterbeds, beanbag chairs, or padded mattresses. Remove all pillows from around your infant, as well as blankets and comforters. Bed sharing by itself neither causes nor prevents SIDS.

Other doctors have strong feelings against cobedding. They believe that this practice creates a dependent relationship in which children will have difficulty learning to calm themselves when they leave the family bed. Further, they believe it sets families up for sleep problems down the road.

Make an Informed Decision

It's important to remember when making choices about cobedding that doctors are often sharing their own personal opinions on this subject. They may not have studied this issue in medical school, and sometimes a doctor's opinion, like anyone's opinion, might have no basis in fact. Ask for current research on best practices, and remember that there are two sides to every issue. Most health care providers remain flexible and offer cobedding as an important option for breastfeeding pairs.

Don't introduce cereal or other solids early just to help your baby sleep through the night. Your baby's digestive system is not mature enough to handle those foods until around four to six months of age.

Talk to other families who have made this choice. Most importantly, talk to your spouse or bed partner. Men sometimes don't like sharing a bed with infants and toddlers. They might be afraid of rolling over onto the baby or they might resent the loss of intimacy. It's also possible that a one time swift kick in the wrong spot will leave your man sleeping in an uncomfortable defensive position.

Many men share a bed with their babies without problem or complaint, but that doesn't mean that a good father should necessarily be willing to cobed. Alternatives to cobedding include having a bassinet at your bedside, purchasing a cosleeping bedding device, or moving the baby's crib into your room. The crib mattress should be tight against your own mattress at the same level without any space between the two. Lock or block the crib wheels to prevent a gap from forming between the mattresses. You might even consider tying the crib frame to your bed frame for a nice, secure fit. You can adjust the crib gate so you can easily pick up your infant for breastfeeding in the middle of the night.

Safety First

Dr. William and Martha Sears state that parents instinctively know not to roll over on their babies. "The same subconscious awareness that keeps you from rolling off the bed keeps you from rolling onto baby." Still, there are precautions you should take.

FACTS

Cobedding does not have to affect your ability to engage in amorous adventures with your spouse. However, you might be inclined to discover new areas of the house. Changing times and places can add an element of surprise to your lovemaking that you both might find exciting.

Make sure that your bed is not overcrowded. Toddlers should not sleep with infants. They thrash in their sleep, often turning sideways in bed without any conscious awareness of it.

Obviously, parents should not use any drugs or alcohol while cobedding with their infants. The risk of suffocation is far greater when a parent is under the influence.

Sudden Infant Death Syndrome

Sudden Infant Death Syndrome (SIDS) is the sudden and unexplainable death of infants from birth through one year of age. More boys than girls are victims, and most deaths happen during the fall, winter, and early spring months.

Fortunately, the SIDS Foundation's Back to Sleep Campaign is one that works. Since its inception ten years ago, there has been a 42 percent decrease in SIDS-related deaths! That's an incredible number of lives saved through prevention.

There is little known about this condition, also known as crib death, that claims the lives of 7,000 babies each year, but the SIDS Foundation has made recommendations about how death from SIDS can be prevented.

Place your baby on her back to sleep on a firm mattress. Infants don't have the head and neck control to maneuver their air space when placed on their tummies, and some research indicates that SIDS is related to rebreathing carbon dioxide. If your baby has a birth defect or has a breathing, heart, or lung condition, or any other special need, talk to your health care provider. While many mothers worry that infants might choke on their spitup, research does not indicate this to be a threat. There is no increase in suffocation-related deaths because of back sleeping.

Do not smoke around your baby, and do not allow others to smoke around your baby. SIDS deaths are more common in families who smoke. In fact, the risks of smoking and cobedding have been correlated with SIDS. Just as you wouldn't smoke in bed for your own health reasons, do not smoke in bed with your baby.

There are times when it's appropriate to place your baby on her stomach, but not at bedtime. Babies need opportunities for tummy time to help develop muscles and skills. When your baby is alert and you are with her, place her on her tummy. This is a great opportunity for infant exercise!

Be sure that your child care provider as well as your baby's alternative caregivers and grandparents follow these important prevention strategies, too! Consistency in care is critical. Babies who are used to sleeping on their backs but are placed on their tummies in another's care are actually at twenty times greater risk for SIDS.

Soft mattresses and pillows pose a hazard because they can fold around your baby's mouth and nose. Avoid the use of frilly, overstuffed comforters, sheepskin, heavy fleece, and bumper pads in your baby's crib. If your baby is wearing a sleeper to bed, she needs only a light blanket. Similarly, don't place stuffed animals, toys, or pillows in your baby's cradle. These, too, are suffocation hazards.

CHAPTER 7

Is This Right? Evaluating Breastfeeding

Most mothers are concerned that they might not have enough milk to nourish their infant. This is a common, but unnecessary, fear. Our uncertainty over our milk supply arises because we like to measure everything scientifically. When you breastfeed, there is no reliable direct method of knowing how much milk your baby receives, but doctors generally follow two guidelines when assessing breastmilk intake: infant weight gain and elimination patterns.

Weight Gain

Infant weight gain is one of the most important indicators of an adequate milk supply. However, it's normal for babies to lose 5 to 8 percent of their birthweight during the first few days of life. After that, babies gain about one ounce of weight per day, and by their two-week checkup, they should surpass their birthweight by a few ounces. A baby who weighs less than her birthweight at her two-week checkup might not be feeding adequately.

FACTS

Too often, parents are concerned when their infant is in the low or high end of the growth chart for their age. Growth charts were developed using formula-fed infants as the baseline, so don't worry if your baby weighs in lower than "normal" on the chart.

Breastfed babies gain weight more rapidly than formula-fed infants during the first two months of life, then slow down around the fourth month. By six months of age, their birthweight should have doubled. If you have concerns about your baby's weight, call your doctor. You can have your baby weighed any time.

Elimination Patterns

The second best indicator of adequate milk intake is frequent bowel movements and urination. What goes in must come out.

Soon after birth, your baby will pass meconium, a thick, sticky, dark substance produced by the liver. After two days, your baby's bowel movements will change to a greenish-brown color and will look like thick pea soup. He will pass two to three stools per day. By day five, your baby's stools will change again, this time to a loose, yellow mustard, cottage cheese, or seedlike consistency. These are called milk stools. Your baby will pass two to five stools per day, most likely during a feeding, or when he's fast asleep and ready to be put down.

Your baby will also wet frequently. During the first two days, he might wet only once or twice. The colostrum you produce is highly digestible and perfect nutrition for your baby, so there's not much left to eliminate. After your abundant milk comes in, your baby will wet five to eight cloth diapers per day, or four to six disposables. With ultra-absorbent diapers on the market, it can be hard to tell how much he has wet. You can lay a Kleenex inside the diaper to help you tell when your baby urinates.

Call your pediatrician if your baby exhibits symptoms of dehydration: lethargy, weak cry, dry mouth, depressed or sunken fontanel (soft spot) on the top of his head, loss of skin resilience (springiness), or fever.

The urine will be pale yellow or colorless and odorless. If it's dark or looks like redbrick dust, it could be a sign that your baby is not getting enough milk. If your baby is wetting frequently but not stooling, he might not be getting enough hindmilk.

If your baby is not passing at least two stools per day and wetting six to eight diapers after his first week of life, he could be on his way to dehydration. This is a very serious health threat for babies. Talk to your pediatrician immediately.

Breast Changes

Your breasts change during pregnancy, then once more with the birth of your baby, and again after a solid nursing routine is established. Lactogenesis leaves breasts full within three to five days postpartum.

Most women produce an ounce of milk per breast per hour. Breasts generally feel full before a feeding and softer afterward, but because breasts don't have fuel gauges, the only surefire way to measure your milk is to express it. Even then, you won't get a true indication of your milk volume. A pump simply cannot remove milk as efficiently as your baby can.

According to infant studies, your baby needs about one to two ounces of milk per feeding per month of age.

Day 1:   5 ccs (colostrum)
Day 2:   15 ccs or ½ ounce (colostrum)
Day 3:   30 ccs or 1 ounce (colostrum)
Day 4:   2 ounces (transitional milk)
Day 5:   2–2½ ounces (transitional milk)

You can also gauge how much your baby needs at each feeding by his weight:

6–8 pounds: 2 ounces
9–12 pounds: 3 ounces
13–15 pounds: 4 ounces
15+ pounds: 5 ounces

As your baby suckles, you might feel a tingling or pins-and-needles sensation that lets you know your milk is letting down. As you nurse your baby, milk leaking from the opposite breast is also a sign that your milk has let down.

QUESTIONS?

What effect, if any, will an epidural during labor have on milk production?
Epidurals used during labor and delivery cause overhydration of body tissues. Overhydration makes it difficult for hormones that stimulate the production of milk, like prolactin, to reach breast cells across this lake of fluid. If you've had an epidural during labor, talk to a lactation consultant before hospital discharge.

Some women don't have these sensations, nor do they observe leakage. If you don't know if your milk has let down, you might need the assistance of a lactation consultant. Stress and fatigue can inhibit the milk ejection reflex, and this can ultimately reduce your milk supply.

Some mothers feel tenderness during their first week of breastfeeding. However, this discomfort usually subsides after the baby has latched on correctly. If you experience sore, cracked, or blistered nipples, your baby is not latching on correctly and might not be adequately removing milk from the breast.

If you have not experienced any change in your breasts during pregnancy or after the birth of your baby, you'll need to have a breast exam performed by your doctor. A rare condition exists in a very few women that affects the growth of their mammary tissues. This under-development inhibits milk production. Women who have had breast reduction surgery or a mastectomy are also at risk for insufficient milk production. If your doctor has determined that you are physically incapable of producing enough milk to nourish your baby, you will be asked to supplement with formula.

BREASTFEEDING EVALUATION CHECKLIST

Does your baby let you know he's hungry?	Yes	No
Do you position your baby chest to breast with you?	Yes	No
Does your baby open his mouth wide to attach?	Yes	No
Does your baby latch on effectively?	Yes	No
Are his lips flanged around your breast?	Yes	No
Does your baby create a tight seal around your breast?	Yes	No
Is your baby's suck rhythmic for five to ten minutes?	Yes	No
Do you see your baby's ear wiggle while he's feeding?	Yes	No
Do you offer both breasts at each feeding?	Yes	No
Do you feel your milk ejection reflex?	Yes	No
Can you feel your uterus contract when nursing?	Yes	No
Are your breasts softer after each feeding?	Yes	No
Is your baby's hunger satisfied after nursing?	Yes	No
Is your baby gaining weight?	Yes	No
Is your baby passing loose/soft stools two to three times daily?	Yes	No
Is your baby wetting at least five to eight diapers five days after birth?	Yes	No

If you've answered no to any of these questions, ask a lactation consultant to observe your baby during a feeding session. Any problem corrected now will ensure a more successful breastfeeding experience.

Supplemental Feeding and Alternative Methods

If your doctor or lactation consultant determines that your baby isn't getting enough milk, they will work with you to increase your milk production. Increasing breastfeeding frequency, feeding from both breasts, and expressing your breastmilk with a double pump can all increase your prolactin levels and help you produce a more abundant supply.

There may be situations that require you to use an alternative feeding method for a short time as you build your milk supply. With the goal of exclusive breastfeeding in mind, practice any of these methods cautiously and only under the guidance of a lactation consultant or pediatrician. Alternative feeding should be used on a temporary basis to correct breastfeeding problems. It's not usually a viable long-term solution, and it's important to get your baby back to the breast as soon as possible.

SUPPLEMENTAL FEEDING DEVICES AND TECHNIQUES		
TYPE	DESCRIPTION	COMMENTS
Cup Feeding	A flexible one- or two-ounce cup is filled with milk and held to baby's lips. The baby is held upright and allowed to lick at the milk.	DO NOT POUR. Baby should not be crying at start.
Spoon Feeding	This method is similar to cup feeding but utilizes a spoon. A small, soft spoon is best. Some special spoons hold larger amounts of milk in a reservoir so feeding isn't interrupted.	Tedious and time-consuming but effective.
Syringe/Eyedropper Feeding	An eyedropper can be used to drip milk into an upright baby's mouth. A syringe can be used in the same way. A syringe with a long tip can be used to feed at the breast.	Periodontal syringes are best; they have a soft tip that won't hurt baby's gums.
Finger Feeding	The tube of a supplemental feeder is held to a clean adult finger. Baby sucks on the finger and gets milk through the tube.	Effective but some babies prefer it to the breast. *(continued)*

TYPE	DESCRIPTION	COMMENTS
Supplemental Nursing System	A supplemental nutrition system is used when baby can latch onto the breast but needs supplemental feeding. Typically, a reservoir of milk is worn around the mom's neck and tubes from it are inserted into baby's mouth as he suckles. Baby gets both milks, from the breast and from the supplementer.	#1 recommended method. Builds Mom's morale. Teaches proper latch on and stimulates milk production.
Haberman Feeder	A special bottle with a long nipple and a valve that rewards any level of suckling	Useful for babies with developmental delays or oral/facial abnormalities.
Standard Bottle	Any variety of the plain old infant bottle.	Leads to nipple confusion and poor suck.

Supplemental Systems

Supplemental nursing systems, like Medela's SNS or Lact-Aid International's Nursing Trainer, consist of a milk reservoir and a short length of very small, clear tubing. The reservoir is worn around a mother's neck from a cord and the tubing is inserted into the baby's mouth as he nurses at the breast. This technique is the method of choice for most lactation professionals as it allows the breast to be stimulated to increase milk production, helps infants learn proper latch, and preserves the breastfeeding relationship.

FIGURE 7-1: Supplemental Nursing System

Supplementers are used with infants who have weak sucks or nipple confusion from supplemental bottle feeding in the hospital. It's also beneficial for mothers who suffer from reduced milk supply. You can make your own supplementer by cutting a hole in the nipple of a bottle. Add expressed milk or formula. Place one end of a small gavage tube (available at a medical supply store) into the hole. Position your baby at your breast in the cradle or football hold. As you support your breast in the C hold, tuck the tube under your thumb, extending it toward the end of your nipple. Latch your baby to your breast and the tube.

As your infant suckles, he not only receives the milk from the reservoir, but he stimulates and extracts milk from your breast at the same time. Carefully adjust the flow rate to match your baby's ability to keep up. You should be able to hear him swallow milk, but the flow should never be fast enough to cause gagging. Use this method under the guidance of a health care professional.

Cup or Spoon Feeding

Supplemental feeding using a cup can be beneficial for a baby who has jaundice, poor elimination patterns, or inadequate latch. Cup feeding reduces nipple confusion from a bottle and allows the infant to lap milk at his own pace. It can be messy, but it's an easy substitution for breastfeeding.

To begin, place a towel around your baby or swaddle him in a blanket. Fill a spoon or a soft, flexible cup half full with expressed milk. Bring the cup or spoon to the baby's lower lip. Drip just enough milk into his mouth to taste. Tip the spoon so your baby can lick the milk. This process is slower than putting baby to the breast but can be used to supplement breastfeeding, as needed. Use of an eyedropper can also be effective.

Finger Feeding

Finger feeding is hard to learn, awkward, and can cause dependency, but it is useful for babies who have a weak suck, nipple confusion, or neurological problems.

Insert a small gavage tube into the nipple of a baby bottle filled with expressed milk. Place your baby in a semireclining position. Offer a clean finger (nail side down) slowly into your baby's mouth, moving it back to the soft palate. If your baby gags, bring you finger forward slightly, and wait until he's comfortable. Place the tube or periodontal syringe next to your finger. As your baby suckles, he will draw milk from the bottle, or you can offer a small squirt from the syringe.

FIGURE 7-2:
Finger
feeding

FIGURE 7-3:
Syringe
feeding

Bottle Feeding

Bottle feeding might be the only alternative available when other techniques don't work. It can be useful for mothers with sore nipples or if an infant can't open his mouth wide enough to latch to the breast. However, many babies who switch from breast to bottle and back again will suffer from nipple confusion. Bottle nipples flow faster than the breast, and once babies develop a dependency on the bottle, they often refuse the breast.

Many parents find that infants accept supplemental feedings more easily from Dad than from Mom. A baby grows comfortable with the breastfeeding relationship she establishes with her mother and can sometimes be confused when her breastfeeding buddy tries to offer a less satisfying alternative. Supplemental and alternative feeding methods give Dad a wonderful opportunity to take part in the feeding of his child. Finger feeding, cup feeding, spoons, bottles, and eyedroppers can be used by anyone. Many fathers enjoy being able to solve problems, and giving supplemental feedings can be a rewarding way to help them feel more connected to their children.

CHAPTER 8
Common Concerns

Sometimes there are challenges when you're breastfeeding. Whether your baby has difficulty latching on or you need to suspend breastfeeding for your own health reasons, anything that interferes with milk removal can diminish your supply. If your baby doesn't take in enough milk, your body won't produce enough milk. Fortunately, most breast-feeding problems are easily resolved if you catch them early enough.

Does Breastfeeding Hurt?

You may experience some temporary discomfort the first week of breastfeeding. Your baby takes your nipple and part of the areola to the back of his mouth, and he compresses the areola to express milk from the sinuses. You should feel a gentle tug that will take some getting used to.

If you do feel actual nipple pain while nursing, your baby might not be positioned correctly. Your nipple has more pain receptors than your areola, so, if your baby is feeding from the nipple, you'll feel it. Continued nipple feeding can lead to cracked or blistered nipples. Break the latch and try again. If everything else seems to be all right but nipple pain persists after a week, check for thrush.

SSENTIALS

Prolonged nipple pain is an indication that something is wrong. Contact your lactation consultant if you experience any kind of pain while nursing your baby.

You might feel some minor breast discomfort with your milk ejection reflex or letdown. Sensations vary from slight tingles to pins and needles. Letdown lasts less than thirty seconds. You'll also feel some breast fullness with engorgement, however this normally decreases within two days.

Engorgement

Engorgement usually happens around three to five days postpartum. Your mature milk comes in, in preparation for exclusive breastfeeding. When engorgement happens, it can be extremely uncomfortable. You wake up one morning with breasts the size of cantaloupes. They're swollen, your nipple and areola are tight, and your baby has little flexible tissue to latch onto. While this lasts only for a couple of days, it can be painful.

Frequent feedings will help reduce engorgement. They will also regulate your milk supply. If your baby has difficulty latching on, express just enough milk to make yourself comfortable and your breasts pliable.

After your baby has had her fill, you can express more milk and either refrigerate or freeze it for later use. (Remember, though, that any milk that is removed will be replaced. That's the law of supply and demand.)

Warm showers will relieve the pressure of engorgement, and your milk will begin to leak naturally. Heat, in general, will soften your breasts. A warm washcloth on full breasts can help to alleviate discomfort.

Cabbage Leaves

Although there is no known medical reason why cabbage leaves should help with engorgement, many mothers and lactation professionals will attest to the fact that they work. Cabbage leaves have been used throughout the centuries in other countries. It's a timeless, yet "new age," method for reducing engorgement.

Cabbage leaves should be used only as long as the discomfort of engorgement lasts. Prolonged use can diminish your milk supply.

Here's what you do: Buy a medium cabbage. Peel and clean the leaves, then store them in Ziploc bags. Refrigerate. When you're ready to use them, select enough leaves to completely cover your breasts on all sides, as well as the area under your armpit. Gently crush the leaves to break the veins, then apply the cool leaves to your breasts. Lie back on a towel and relax, or tuck them securely into your bra. The cool cabbage leaves will help reduce the pain and swelling associated with engorgement.

Within two hours, you'll begin to feel relief. Some milk might leak, so if you're using the bra method, line your bra with nursing pads or other absorbent materials. You should reapply new leaves after two hours, or whenever they appear wilted.

Other Comfort Measures

Although the engorgement phase is relatively brief, you'll want to give yourself every advantage to ensure your comfort until your nursing routine is established. In addition to cool cabbage leaves and warm showers, consider the following suggestions:

- Wear a supportive bra.
- Take ibuprofen (Motrin, Nuprin, or Advil) for pain.
- Wrap a plastic bag of ice chips or frozen vegetables in a washcloth. (Peas or corn work best because of their size, but you can use whatever is available.) The bag will conform to the shape of your breast and can be used for fifteen to twenty minutes of relief. If you plan to refreeze the bag of vegetables and use it again later, mark it as inedible. Repeated freezing and thawing promotes the growth of bacteria.
- A refrigerated rice sock works wonders, too. Rice socks are used by doulas to relieve pain during labor. They conform to your body and provide relief by interrupting the pain receptors that carry messages to the brain. Rice socks can be heated or cooled. To cool, toss it in the freezer for an hour. To heat, toss it in the microwave for thirty seconds at a time (for up to two minutes). When using the microwave method, carefully shake the sock so the heat is evenly distributed. Wrap the rice sock in a washcloth or sheet to protect your skin.

FACTS

To make your own rice sock, fill a clean cotton tube sock with plain white rice. Add a drop of your favorite aromatherapy scent, like lavender, for relaxation. Sew the top closed with a needle and thread. Rice socks can be used over and over again, but they cannot be washed. They last a long time and can be used to relieve aches and pains in daily life (sore muscles, headaches, cramps).

Remember that this stage is only temporary. Try any combination of the relief methods until the discomfort passes and you and your baby can have a comfortable breastfeeding session.

Leaking

Many women have concerns that their milk will leak during business presentations or while out in public. It can happen. However, some women don't experience any leaking at all. Leaking most often occurs during the first few weeks of lactation and usually only continues with women who have a very abundant milk supply. There are exceptions, of course, and leaking or even spraying milk during lovemaking is common.

If you experience frequent leaking:

- Nurse your baby frequently, especially before going out or making love.
- Use absorbent cotton breastpads or cloths to catch the drips.
- Place bath towels under you when in bed.
- Press your folded arms gently against your chest to draw your breasts into your body.

There are occasions when you'll experience letdown at the thought or smell of your baby. A crying child in the supermarket might even turn on your milk like a faucet. Generally, though, most women who feed their babies regularly won't leak after a breastfeeding routine is well established.

Sore Nipples and Blisters

Sore nipples are usually a sign of nipple feeding or improper latch. When babies feed only on the nipple, nipples can crack and blister. Blisters also occur as a result of rubbing against the roof of baby's mouth or along his gums. The pain associated with a blistered nipple can make nursing very uncomfortable, but it's important to continue breastfeeding.

Sometimes cracked nipples bleed, but that doesn't have to interfere with nursing. A little bit of your blood, mixed with your milk, will not harm your baby.

To treat sore nipples:

- Ensure that your baby has a good latch. (Wait until he opens wide, then grasp him to the breast, pointing your nipple to the roof of his mouth. He needs to take in an inch of the areola as well.)
- Use different nursing positions to vary the way your baby latches onto your nipple.
- Offer the least tender breast first so that your milk will let down in the other breast without your baby creating suction.
- Express your milk using a pump to help your milk let down before offering your breast to your baby.
- Break suction evenly by inserting your finger into your baby's mouth. (Don't allow your baby to slide off your nipple.)
- Apply lanolin to a sore nipple. (Like chapped lips, nipples heal more quickly with moisture. You don't need to remove modified lanolin before your baby nurses.)
- Use breast shells to keep your nipples from rubbing against fabric.

Remember, also, to avoid using soap on your nipples. The Montgomery glands produce natural oils to clean and protect your nipples; soap may aggravate the situation by drying them out further.

Plugged Ducts

Plugged milk ducts occur when there is an insufficient removal of milk from the breast. The retained milk forms a cheeselike blockage in the duct, causing a small lump that might be painful, red, or swollen. If neglected, plugged ducts can lead to infections.

The best way to prevent a plugged duct is simply to breastfeed as often as your baby wants, making sure that he finishes one breast before starting another. It's also helpful to change nursing positions. Different positions help your baby remove the milk from all of the ducts. Finally, be sure to wear a comfortable bra. Avoid anything that binds or constrains the breasts, including underwires.

If one of your ducts does become plugged, check for a plugged nipple. Milk residue can sometimes dry in a nipple pore, forming a blockage. If you see a small white dot, like a whitehead, on your nipple, you might have a plugged pore. Nipple blockages are often removed by your baby's suckling. They can also be removed by your health care provider, although many women find that careful work with a fingernail does the trick.

If no nipple blockage is apparent:

- Apply a warm cloth to the affected area for fifteen to twenty minutes before each feeding.
- Nurse more frequently, beginning each session with the affected breast.
- Massage the breast near the plugged duct as your baby nurses or in a warm shower, gently working from behind the plug toward the nipple.

When the plug breaks loose, you might see a filament of solidified milk. It looks like a string and can be several inches in length. If you see one of these strings in your baby's mouth after nursing, don't be alarmed. It's soft and safe to eat, and it won't choke your baby.

Mastitis

Mastitis is the word doctors use to describe an infection of the breast. These bacterial infections generally begin with a plugged duct or a cracked nipple. A mother with mastitis usually has flu-like symptoms along with a fever and a hard spot or lump in the breast accompanied by pain, redness, and swelling. Mastitis is often treated with antibiotics. Other measures include warm showers, lots of bed rest and fluids, and frequent nursing. The infection is not harmful to babies and is only aggravated by weaning.

Anytime mastitis symptoms last beyond two days or a breast lump remains, you should suspect an abscess. A breast abscess is a pool of pus within the breast tissue. The fluid must be drained by your doctor.

Recovery is rapid after draining, but temporary weaning from the infected breast might be required.

Thrush

Thrush or candida is another name for a common yeast infection of both mothers and babies. Most children with candida became infected as they passed through the birth canal. The first symptoms usually occur in two to four weeks. On occasion, babies become infected much later, usually after the use of antibiotics. If you've nursed comfortably for many weeks or months but are suddenly experiencing pain, thrush might be the problem.

Infants with thrush have white patches inside their mouths or an angry rash on their bottoms. Mothers often have sharp, shooting pains in their breasts, and sometimes red, tender nipples or patches of red or white on the breast.

Thrush can be very painful, but it responds well to treatment. Doctors typically prescribe an antifungal rinse for baby's mouth and an antifungal cream or ointment for baby's bottom (boy or girl) and mother's nipples. However, medication alone is not always effective. In addition to medical treatment, you should:

- Rinse the affected breasts and diaper area with clean water and let them air dry.
- Expose the affected area to the sun for a few minutes, once or twice per day.
- Change your nursing pads after every feeding session.
- Change diapers frequently—yeast thrives in warm, damp places.
- Wash bras, bottle nipples, breast shells, pacifiers, and any other items that come into contact with the infected areas in hot, soapy water.
- Use lanolin or other breastfeeding-friendly nipple treatments to relieve pain.
- Wash your hands before and after each feeding or treatment.
- Drink more water and eat less sugar.
- Treat your partner if he has had contact with your breasts.

Many mothers successfully treat thrush with a nonprescription medication called gentian violet. Most pharmacies carry a 1 percent solution of gentian violet that can be applied to all infected areas with a cotton swab, twice daily for three days. It's a pretty color, but it stains everything it comes in contact with, so be careful with your clothing.

If you are expressing milk while you have a yeast infection, pump and dump. Freezing does not kill yeast and stored milk can reinfect your baby.

Nipple Confusion

If your baby has been fed from a bottle, he might find it difficult to feed from the breast. Similarly, a baby who's been exclusively breastfed can find the transition to a bottle difficult. Feeding from a bottle is different from breastfeeding. The suck is different. The volume and flow of milk are different. The taste, texture, and temperature are different. Perhaps most importantly, bottles reward lazy nursing and breasts don't.

When your baby doesn't know how to suckle the breast properly because of bottle or pacifier use, it's called nipple confusion. Nipple confusion threatens your breastfeeding success by compromising your milk production. Your infant's disorganized suck won't effectively remove the milk from your breast. That leads to a decreased milk supply, which leads many moms to supplement nursings with a bottle of formula. However, you need a hungry baby's eager suckling to maintain your milk production.

ESSENTIALS   Because nipple confusion impairs breastfeeding success, new moms should avoid giving their infants bottles or pacifiers for at least the first six weeks of life.

Whether you're transitioning your child from breast to bottle or bottle to breast, be patient and persistent. Your baby will make the change, but it might not happen on the first attempt. The best time to try a new feeding method is when your baby is awake and alert but not too hungry. Your baby will only be frustrated by the change if he's already fussing for dinner. The quiet-alert stage right after he wakes is best.

If you're going from bottle to breast, express some milk before you begin to trigger your letdown reflex. Babies who are used to bottles want their milk immediately. After your baby has caught on to breastfeeding, you can continue nursing him without any special preparation.

If you're transitioning from the breast to a bottle, you might need to experiment with a number of different nipple styles and materials to find one your child likes (see Chapter 13). There are quite a few varieties available, and babies definitely do have individual preferences. Start the move to bottle feeding with expressed breastmilk, but let Dad or another caregiver do the feeding. Some babies simply refuse to take a bottle from Mom when they know there's a perfectly good breast available.

Breastmilk Jaundice

Newborn jaundice is caused by the normal breakdown of excessive red blood cells into bilirubin, a substance that turns babies' tissues yellow. Breastmilk jaundice is different from other jaundice in that it usually occurs in well-fed babies who are older than seven days, and it can persist for many weeks. Some doctors believe that breastmilk contains an unknown substance that lets babies absorb an excessive amount of bilirubin, but don't let that theory scare you.

There is nothing wrong with your milk. The usual course of treatment is to monitor your baby's blood and wait for this normal, physiological process to end. Nurse often. Your baby's body eliminates bilirubin through her stools. The greater the frequency of bowel movements, the quicker the excess bilirubin leaves the body.

QUESTIONS?

What can you do to preserve your milk supply while using alternate feeding methods?
Pump your breasts frequently to maintain your milk supply while your baby is taking formula. Ask about finger feeding or other methods to help reduce nipple confusion while your baby takes formula.

If phototherapy is advised, use a bilirubin blanket. These blankets have fiber-optic lights built in so you can hold and nurse your baby while she receives her treatment. Occasionally, doctors recommend that a child be given formula instead of breastmilk for twelve to twenty-four hours. This quickly lowers the bilirubin levels in baby's bloodstream. However, even one day of bottle feeding can interfere with your breastfeeding success.

Teething and Biting

If and when your baby bites your nipple (and after you've regained consciousness), firmly tell her "No" and break the latch. Look her in the eye and tell her "No biting." Be serious but not angry. She may already be in tears after your surprised reaction. Offer the breast again, but if she continues to bite, give her a teething toy to help reinforce its use. Offer expressed milk, water, or juice in a sippy cup to complete the feeding and try breastfeeding again later. Soon, your baby will begin to associate biting with the items you have offered, but your consistency is key.

Do not offer a teething infant anything chokable to help teeth erupt. Ice cubes and many frozen foods can easily lead to tragedy. Raw vegetables and hard fruits will have to wait until baby has lots of teeth to chew them.

Luckily, teething begins around six months of age (depending in part on heredity), so most babies are beginning solids. However, some babies are born with a tooth, called a milk tooth, so learning to get around this little dental ditty happens much earlier.

What if your baby refuses the breast because of teething pain? Again, try the cup. Or call your pediatrician about using an over-the-counter infant teething gel. Your little darling might accept the breast more readily if her gums are numbed. You want to ensure that she's receiving adequate nutrition, so offer chilled mashed bananas, expressed breastmilk, or cold 100 percent natural, unsweetened applesauce.

A Teething Primer

You won't find any hard-and-fast rules on how long it takes a baby to cut his teeth. Every baby is unique and tooth development happens at different rates, but it generally takes two weeks to two months once the tooth is near the surface of the swollen gum.

The pressure of biting helps relieve the pain of teething. Your baby is not being mean when he bites you; he is just doing what comes naturally. As you begin to notice signs that your baby is teething, develop a strategy. Offer him frozen teething rings; a wet, cool washcloth; a feeding spoon; a sippy cup lid; or a pacifier. Cold will help numb his gums, while biting works the teeth through the gums.

Teething and Nipple Care

On occasion, a baby breaks the skin on his mother's nipple with a bite. More commonly, teething will chap the nipple due to increased acids in the saliva or as a result of baby's teeth rubbing against the nipple. Use your breastmilk to coat the nipple and let it air dry. If your injury is severe, your doctor will recommend a safe antibiotic ointment for use between nursing sessions so bacteria doesn't cause infection. This will need to be washed off before you nurse your baby. Moist healing is preferred for nipple care and treatment.

Lack of Support

Many new moms are understandably nervous about breastfeeding their babies. You've probably heard stories from family or friends who tried to breastfeed their babies but gave up. "I couldn't produce enough milk," is the most common reason moms give for abandoning nursing in favor of bottle feeding.

Often, the real cause in these cases was a lack of confidence and support. New moms who aren't sure their baby is getting enough milk through nursing might be tempted to use formula. However, your breasts make only enough milk to supply your baby's demands. If you worry that you're not producing enough milk and offer formula, the amount of milk you produce decreases from a lack of demand. Then, you're in a downward spiral. Less milk means more formula, which means less demand until, pretty soon, you've shut down altogether—all from lack of confidence.

SSENTIALS Reassure bottle-feeding moms that they are good mothers, but if nothing works with the critics, surround yourself with positive voices instead. Get together with women who nursed successfully or join a lactation support group like La Leche League. Remember, you can do it!

A good lactation consultant or pediatrician can help you be successful. So can your husband, family, and friends. Unfortunately, there will be people who aren't supportive of your decision to breastfeed and they can undermine your breastfeeding experience. Sometimes husbands aren't too thrilled about sharing your breasts with a baby. Even other women might be defensive about your decision to breastfeed, especially if they bottle fed their own children. This might include your own mother or mother-in-law. When you talk about the virtues of breastfeeding, they might feel a need to justify bottle feeding. Try to keep their fears in mind when they criticize your decision to nurse.

CHAPTER 9
Colic

Breastmilk is the best food for your child, and breastfeeding is the most comforting way she can get it. Still, colic can threaten your breast-feeding experience. Feelings of frustration and disappointment don't exactly leave you wanting to be close to your baby, much less nurse her, but there are things you can do to get through the experience and come out of it as a strong breast-feeding pair.

What Is Colic?

Crying is a very powerful tool! It is your baby's most effective means of communication. Babies cry for many different reasons. They cry when they're hungry. They cry when they're wet or have a dirty diaper. They cry when they feel scared, lonely, or hurt. They even cry when they're bored. Within the first two weeks of your baby's life, you will learn to distinguish between your baby's different cries. You'll even be able to distinguish her cries from others in a roomful of babies!

Whenever your child cries, you know something is wrong and you instinctively come to her aid. Usually, you can find the problem quickly. You pick up your baby, check her diaper, reassure her, and perhaps offer her a breast. When nothing seems to work, lay people will call it colic. Pediatricians are a little more precise, but not much. They usually consider a baby to be colicky if she follows the rule of three: She cries continuously for three or more hours, three or more times each week, for three or more weeks.

FACTS

Between 10 percent and 15 percent of newborns suffer from colic. Symptoms usually begin within a few weeks of birth and last from three to four months. There are many theories, but no general agreement as to its cause.

The word colic is really a catchall for any condition that causes inconsolable crying and screaming in infants. Colicky babies are in pain. Often, their tummies are hard and distended. They arch their backs, ball their fists, flail their arms and legs, and generally have a hard time with everything from nursing to sleeping. Most babies will calm down when put to the breast and fall asleep shortly after feeding, but not a colicky baby. A colicky baby is more likely to suck vigorously for just a few minutes and then pull away screaming and struggling.

Fussiness versus Colic

It's important not to confuse colic with ordinary fussiness. Crying infants are difficult to feed and do not breastfeed effectively. Fussy infants can be consoled at the breast. Most colicky infants cannot.

Every baby will have periods of fussiness, especially during the first few weeks of life. Not only are they new to the world, but the world is new to them. It's louder, colder, and brighter than the womb, and it can take some getting used to.

QUESTIONS?

Is there a way to differentiate between colic and fussiness? Standard fussiness seems to follow predictable patterns. Crying often peaks with babies in their second week of life. They cry more frequently and with more intensity because of environmental overstimulation and growth spurts.

Like adults, every baby has a different temperament, and some are naturally more demanding and sensitive than others. Think of these high-maintenance babies as having especially sharp senses. Gas pain that wouldn't upset most babies can be very distressing to one with more delicate sensibilities.

Growth Spurts and Temperament

Babies experience growth spurts around two to three weeks and again at six weeks. During these times, your baby might fuss because she is hungry. You're making enough milk, it's just time to take production up another notch. Your baby is growing and prepping your body for the additional nourishment she needs.

Babies experiencing growth spurts tend to feed more often, especially during the evening. After several cluster feeds, your baby will doze off for several hours. Because your milk supply is lower in the evening, your baby can cluster feed without developing gastritis.

Letting your baby nurse more often will quickly increase your milk supply and satisfy her appetite. If you are returning to work during this time, frequent pumping is important.

What Causes Colic?

Because there is no single condition described by the word colic, there really is no single cause. Immature digestive and nervous systems are often thought to be at the root of colic simply because babies seem to miraculously grow out of it by four months of age, a time when those systems have become significantly more developed. For some babies, many different factors can come into play.

One common cause of colic is food allergy. Tiny particles of food, called allergens, find their way from your body into your breastmilk. Some of these allergens simply irritate your baby's intestinal lining. Others leak through that lining and enter your baby's bloodstream, causing her immune system to respond. The typical symptoms of a food allergy in infants are rashes, gas, discolored and mucousy stools, vomiting, a stuffy nose, a red ring around the anus, or a refusal to nurse.

If your baby makes frequent clicking or slurping sounds at the breast, suspect a poor seal between the breast and her mouth, or that her tongue is out of position. Poor latch will allow your baby to swallow air, increasing the chances of an upset stomach and gas pains.

Another cause of colic is gastroesophageal reflux, or GER. Basically, GER is a condition in which immature development of a muscular valve at the intersection of the stomach and the esophagus lets stomach acid enter your child's esophagus. The acid causes a painful sensation like heartburn. Babies who spit up a lot and fail to gain weight are often diagnosed with GER. This is a serious condition and must be monitored by your health care provider. Breastfed babies are three times less likely to have GER than formula-fed babies.

The other typical causes of colic have to do with the way your baby nurses. Too much milk letdown too quickly causes a baby to take big gulps of air, leading to an upset stomach. Air can also be swallowed if your baby's mouth doesn't form a tight seal around the breast. Some of the latest research on colic and nursing has shown that some babies might become colicky when they switch from breast to breast too soon and fill up on foremilk. Foremilk is very lactose-rich and the excess lactose can ferment in your baby's body, causing gas, bloating, and explosive, greenish stools. This doesn't mean your baby is lactose-intolerant. It just means he's getting too much foremilk.

How Long Will This Last?

No one can say with certainty how long a baby (and her parents) will suffer from colic. Some babies suffer for months, while others recover in a few days. The same is true regarding the timing and duration of a particular episode of colicky screaming. Some babies cry only at certain times of the day, and others scream inconsolably day and night.

Eventually, whatever it is gets better. Most children recover from colic by the beginning of their fourth month of life. Historically, people called colic in newborns "three-month colic," indicating an awareness of that wonderful fourth month. Even food allergies and the heartburnlike pain of GER will pass. By six months of age, your baby's intestines will be mature enough to handle most food proteins that are present in your breastmilk. Within the next six months, the muscular valve at the top of your baby's stomach will have developed enough to prevent GER.

What Can I Do?

The first thing to do if your baby shows symptoms of colic is to eliminate all the normal causes of fussiness. Respond quickly to her cries. Offer the breast. Provide any physical security she might need.

If your baby can't be consoled, make an appointment with your pediatrician right away. Doctors typically use a diagnosis of colic when a baby seems healthy and is gaining weight but can't be consoled. Insist that your child's health care provider make a reasonable effort to find the problem.

A diagnosis of GER gives you a chance to reduce both the frequency and the severity of colic attacks. As always, breast is best. Your milk digests more rapidly than formula in your baby's stomach, so there's less chance for stomach contents to back up into the esophagus. Doctors recommend that feedings be frequent and small. Propping up the head of the crib is also helpful in keeping stomach acid down.

Babies with GER often sleep best on their stomachs, but stomach sleeping has been associated with an increased risk of SIDS, also known as crib death. Follow the advice of your health care provider.

The same day you see the doctor, see your lactation specialist. She'll need to observe a normal breastfeeding session. She'll check the seal between baby's mouth and your breast, and will observe the amount of time your baby spends on each breast as well as whether letdown is overwhelming your baby.

If your baby is swallowing air, there are solutions. Check your nursing posture and the feeding position of your baby, and make her open her mouth wide before you let her take the breast.

If you suspect your baby isn't nursing long enough on each breast to get hindmilk, remember to let her nurse as long as she wants before switching sides. Don't feel that you need to move her to the second breast after some predetermined amount of time. Clocks can't tell you when to switch sides. Both your breasts and your baby will quickly adjust to this change in the feeding pattern.

If your baby seems to quit nursing before your letdown occurs, try breast compression to get her interested again. Breast compression is very much like manual milk expression (see Chapter 12), except that you do it while your baby still has your breast in her mouth.

Food Review

After you've eliminated medical causes and nursing problems from your list of suspects, take a look at your diet. Most women can eat anything they want while breastfeeding and never experience any problems. A few of us aren't so lucky.

However, an actual food allergy isn't necessary for a food to cause problems for your child. Any baby can react to something you've eaten. Some foods might bother your baby by causing gas or irritating her intestinal lining. The best way to check for food sensitivities is to systematically remove suspect foods from your diet and watch for changes in your baby's symptoms.

If someone in your family has food allergies, your child is more likely to be sensitive to stray food proteins in your breastmilk. You might even be allergic to a food yourself and not realize it.

There are certain foods that seem to cause colic symptoms more than others, but every breastfeeding woman and every nursing child is unique. Consider any list of "problem" foods to be nothing more than a convenient starting point for your tests.

Once you've identified a food that seems to cause a reaction in your baby, eliminate it from your diet. Most foods will clear from your body within forty-eight hours, but it may be a week or so before the last traces of some foods are gone. During that transitional time, your baby's colic might continue. Hang in there and remember that colic can be caused by a combination of things, so eliminating a problem food can often be just the first step.

You might find yourself really missing a favorite food, but don't worry. It's only temporary. If you're brave and have nerves of steel, you might try the food again in tiny amounts on rare occasions. Some babies seem to be able to tolerate that kind of exposure. Otherwise, wait a few months before reintroducing the offending food to your diet. As your baby grows, her intestinal tract matures enough to handle food proteins in your milk, and many allergies will fade away.

PROBLEM FOODS: THE USUAL SUSPECTS*

INGREDIENT	REACTION
Caffeine	Because very young infants can't eliminate caffeine from their bodies very well, it can build up in their system and make them irritable. Caffeine is present in chocolate, soft drinks, coffee, tea, and some cold medicines.
Chocolate	Theobromine, a chemical found in chocolate, irritates the lining of a baby's stomach, resulting in fussiness or diarrhea.
Citrus fruits	Oranges, grapefruits, lemons, and limes can irritate a baby's stomach and intestines. Symptoms include sniffles, diarrhea, skin rashes, fussiness, hives, or vomiting.
Cow's milk	Dairy products are the most common cause of allergic reactions in infants. Symptoms can include cough, diarrhea, fussiness, gas, rash, runny nose, or congestion.
Eggs, wheat, corn, fish, nuts, soy	These foods can pass into your milk and cause diarrhea, skin rashes, hives, sniffles, fussiness, or vomiting.
Gassy vegetables	Cauliflower, onion, garlic, cabbage, broccoli, peppers, cucumbers, and turnips can cause gas and fussiness, especially when eaten raw.
Spicy foods	Spicy foods probably cause problems simply by changing the flavor of your milk or, rarely, by irritating your baby's stomach. The only symptom is usually a refusal to nurse.

*Medicines and iron supplements are also commonly blamed for colic.

Sound

Your vacuum cleaner is about to become your new best friend. The sound of a vacuum has been known to instantly calm a colicky baby. Get out the Hoover and give it a try. If you can't use the vacuum cleaner, tune the television to a static-filled channel and turn up the volume. Other good sources of white noise are detuned radios or small appliances like blenders and mixers. You can even buy the sounds of your child's favorite appliances on tape or CD for use away from the home.

Another calming sound for many babies is music. Since it worked for the Tasmanian Devil, it's worth a try for your colicky baby. If you played a particular piece of music during pregnancy or you often sing to your child, those songs might help her relax. If not, experiment with different types of music. The one that works might not be your favorite style, but you'll soon learn to love it out of sheer gratitude.

FACTS

You might be tempted to just forget about breastfeeding and switch to formula, but that can be a major mistake. Most babies who have a food allergy are sensitive to cows' milk, the primary ingredient in baby formula. Instead of eliminating colic, formula may actually make it worse.

Don't underestimate the power of your own voice cooing softly in your baby's ear. Use your voice as an instrument. Sing. Change tones. Babies respond well to "parentese," that higher-pitched tone moms and dads often use when speaking to infants.

Movement

Movement is soothing to all babies. Anyone who has ever cared for a crying child knows that rocking, bouncing, or the gentle vibrations of a moving vehicle can lull a baby into sleep. Calming movement seems instinctive when you try to soothe your child. Most parents have tried rocking and gently bouncing their baby in their arms, but don't stop there. Try dancing, moving from side to side, baby swings, and bouncy chairs. Movement is often more effective when combined with some of the other techniques. Placing your baby in her car seat on top of a running clothes dryer provides gentle movement and white noise at the same time. (If you do try the dryer approach, be sure both your baby and her seat are secure.)

Never shake your baby! Shaken baby syndrome has claimed the lives of countless newborns. Colic is frustrating for both parent and infant. If you feel like you're on your last nerve, call a friend, family member, or crisis line immediately. Or call Shaken Baby Syndrome Prevention Plus at 1-800-852-5222.

Some movements help your baby expel painful gas. Try putting gentle pressure on your infant's tummy, or try the colic hold. Put your baby facedown along the length of your arm. Her head goes off to one side of your arm at the inner bend of the elbow. Her arms and legs dangle on either side of your forearm, and your hand cups her bottom. Your other hand can then rub her back as you walk or bop in place. This hold takes a lot of strength, so it can be a good reason to hand off your crying baby to your partner for a while.

FIGURE 9-1:
Colic hold

The colic hold places gentle pressure on your baby's tummy, which may ease digestive pains. Combine this hold with rhythmic motions and soothing sounds to help keep you and your baby calm.

A variation on the colic hold turns the baby around on your arm (with her head toward your palm) and lets your other arm come up underneath to help support the baby's weight.

Warm Bath

Some parents have found that taking a colicky baby into a tub of warm water will calm her. This is not only great therapy for your child, it's wonderfully relaxing for you. At the first sign of colic, you both get into the bath and stay there. You might be there all morning or half the night. Just keep adding warm water along the way and nursing when you need to. Lay your baby on your chest, tuck her knees to her tummy, and cover her with a warm washcloth. Gently and continuously cup warm water over her back. The moist heat and skin-to-skin contact have been known to work wonders. Washing your baby with a gentle, scented cleanser enhances the relaxing effects of the bath with a combination of aromatherapy and massage. Lavender is a calming scent for both of you.

Although a warm bath can provide a welcome break from the symptoms of colic for your baby, parents need to take extreme caution with this approach. A tired mom or dad in the bath can easily fall asleep and an infant could drown.

The use of aromatherapy in childhood can lead to a lifetime of relaxation. Nothing brings back a memory like the smells associated with an event. Think about your grandmother's kitchen at Thanksgiving or the smell of a vinyl Barbie doll on Christmas morning. The soft sweetness of the lavender that calms your colicky child now will probably become associated with a feeling of relief and relaxation for the rest of her life.

Swaddling

Swaddling is a way of snugly wrapping your infant in a blanket. This technique sometimes helps to calm a colicky baby. Swaddling keeps her warm and secure, like a cloth hug. It's also a way to keep her from being upset by the way her own body suddenly jerks when she's startled. Swaddled babies often sleep longer and fuss less.

During early infancy, most babies are swaddled from the neck down. Your baby might prefer to have her arms free. Try it both ways. Older babies, however, are generally frustrated by swaddling. If your child is learning to roll or crawl, it's probably time to quit.

Slings

Slings have been used for centuries by mothers in other cultures to keep their babies close to their bodies for warmth, protection, and transportation. Slings act as "transitional wombs." Your baby is close to your breast, can hear your heartbeat, and grows in sync with your body rhythms. Dads who carry their babies in slings bond more quickly as both learn to read each other's cues and movements. Babywearing meets an infant's need for sensory stimulation. Constant contact with their caregivers promotes happier, healthier babies, and studies indicate that sling-carried infants cry less frequently than other babies.

Infant Massage

Massage can often bring a measure of relief to a colicky baby. It can help your baby's body release trapped gas by pushing gas and fecal matter through the intestines to the bowel. Massage also promotes the normal functioning of the intestines, stimulates nervous system development, and provides an opportunity for mother and child to work together in a relaxing and bonding way.

The specific techniques used to massage a colicky baby tend to focus on the abdominal area. Try this:

1. Find a warm, quiet place.
2. Sit on the floor with your back straight and your legs in front of you. Your knees should be bent out to the sides, and your heels should touch.
3. Place your baby on a soft blanket on the floor within the area between your legs.
4. Relax.
5. Ask your baby if she wants a massage. This will serve as her cue that you're about to begin.
6. Remove baby's clothes and diaper. Talk to her about what you're doing.
7. Stroke gently with your hands, palm down on baby's stomach, one hand after the other.
8. Hold your baby's legs up by the ankles with your left hand and continue using scooping strokes on her stomach with your right hand.
9. Put baby's legs down and lay your thumbs flat at her navel. Push out to the sides with the flats of your thumbs. Don't poke.

10. Repeat steps seven to nine six times.
11. Hold your baby's knees together and gently but firmly push them into her stomach. Hold them there for thirty seconds.
12. Gently release your baby's legs and put both hands, palm down, on her stomach. Your right hand should be above your left hand.
13. As your left hand makes a circle moving clockwise, your right hand makes a half-circle in the same direction. A clockwise motion is important because that's the direction food and gas flow in the intestines.
14. Repeat steps twelve to thirteen six times, followed again by step eleven.

When massaging your baby, use a light natural oil (like vegetable oil), not lotion. Baby oil has petroleum products that can seep into baby's skin. Keep all of your motions gentle, long, slow, and rhythmic.

Continue Nursing

Your milk is giving your baby everything she needs to get through this difficult time. As a nursing mother, it might comfort you to know that you can offer your baby a few moments of relief at your breast. If at some point you feel that you just can't do it anymore, express your milk and bottle feed it to your baby.

Coping with a Colicky Infant

The stress caused by a screaming baby, combined with a new parent's lack of confidence and lack of sleep, can take a huge toll on your health and self-esteem. A baby with colic puts a tremendous strain on a family, especially on a nursing mother. It's not uncommon for women to feel disappointed and even angry about their colicky child. Remember that it's not your baby's fault. She's not crying because she is "spoiled." She's simply in pain. There's no such thing as a spoiled infant.

Many colicky babies have their crying jags in the evening when you're already worn out from the day's activities, so sleep whenever you can.

Always good advice to new parents, it's incredibly important for parents of a colicky baby. One of you can take the baby to a far corner of the house or on a long drive while the other naps. Fathers need to step up during colic attacks and offer relief to their breastfeeding partners whenever they can.

FACTS

A colicky baby does not make you a bad parent. It also doesn't mean there's anything wrong with your breastmilk or your genetics. There seems to be no common thread connecting colicky infants, not birth order, culture, class, gender, or anything that happened during pregnancy or birth. Colic just happens.

Over time, the screaming and crying can really wear you and your partner down and deflate your excitement about being parents. Every expectant couple has a dream about what it's going to be like when the baby finally arrives. We all envision an "easy" baby, a baby that's sweet and loving and even fun. The reality is that the arrival of a new baby is a huge change for the entire family. On a scale of one to ten, a "normal" baby changes your life by about nine and a colicky baby changes it by about a thousand.

Don't get trapped into feeling like you have to be there for your baby every minute of every day. A stressed-out, exhausted parent is probably more of a threat to a child's well-being than colic ever could be. Take care of yourself as well as your baby. Watch out for signs of depression and sleep deprivation.

When colic threatens to overwhelm you, express a bottle of breastmilk and get away for a while. Give the baby to your partner and go somewhere special, just for you. Remember that colic is only temporary. Your entire family can get through this and move on to the truly wonderful times that lay ahead for all of you.

CHAPTER 10
Special Circumstances

No food can help your baby grow strong and develop intellectually as well as the milk your body produces naturally. That's especially true when your baby faces challenges others don't. Your body will respond to your baby's special needs with special breastmilk. Sometimes, breastfeeding your baby won't be easy, but if you stay with it, the rewards for the entire family will make it all worthwhile.

Premature Infants

Preemies are often unable to nurse because of medical interventions and their inability to coordinate a sucking pattern. They are also often fed through a gavage tube that's inserted through the mouth and into the stomach. Human milk is the food of choice for fragile infants. The incredible power of your milk, which is specially developed for your premature infant, will help your baby gain weight. It will also protect him in his already compromised state. Your baby will develop more quickly and be less susceptible to infections when he gets your milk, and you'll feel more connected to him and confident in your abilities as a mother.

What You Can Do

Mothers of premature infants are advised to begin using a hospital-grade breast pump as soon as practical after delivery. Frequent pumping will ensure a good milk supply, regardless of how well your baby can latch or suckle. Try to express milk every two to three hours. Every little bit helps, so don't worry about volume at first. Initially, you'll produce just a few drops of colostrum, but that's enough. Colostrum is powerful stuff.

With any baby in a special circumstance, the advice and support of a lactation consultant can make all the difference. At the same time, support groups like La Leche give you access to other women who've successfully met the same challenges that you and your child face.

Let the hospital staff know that you'll provide your milk for all of your baby's feedings. Leave instructions that your expressed milk should be given to your premature baby with a syringe or a spoon. Finger feeding is another method that sometimes works well.

With the help of a qualified lactation consultant, begin breastfeeding your premature infant as soon as possible. Preemies are small, so pump before you begin. A taut, full breast is hard to fit into a tiny mouth.

Pumping also stimulates your letdown reflex, something a preemie's weak suck might have trouble accomplishing on its own.

If you are unable to breastfeed exclusively, you can be fitted with a supplemental feeding device, like a supplemental nutrition system (see Chapter 7). After the baby is attached to the breast, a small tube from the supplementer is inserted into his mouth to provide expressed breastmilk. He learns how to breastfeed and at the same time stimulates the breast to continue milk production.

ESSENTIALS

Sometimes, the positioning of a small newborn is difficult. Because their muscles might be underdeveloped, many women find the football, or clutch, hold useful. The football hold helps because it gives you control and support of your child's head and body.

Preemies have special needs that only your breastmilk can meet. Breastmilk-fed preemies have been shown to enjoy better general health than formula-fed babies. When you give birth prematurely, your breasts produce a special milk, called preterm, that's higher in calories, proteins, and fats to help your baby grow quickly. This superior food for your infant is something that only you can provide.

Kangaroo Care

If your baby was born prematurely or at low birthweight, kangaroo care is a wonderful alternative to incubators. Allowing moms to provide this uniquely tender care, even to babies who are still on respirators, has had some amazing results! Babies who receive kangaroo care:

- Have more regular heartbeats
- Suffer from less sleep apnea
- Are more able to regulate their body temperature
- Gain weight more rapidly
- Sleep better
- Are more successful at breastfeeding

With kangaroo care, the baby is held skin-to-skin on his mother's chest, between her breasts and under her shirt or robe. The baby is kept warm, he can hear the heartbeat and breathing he heard in the womb, and he has instant access to the breast. Most health care providers recommend that periods of kangaroo care should last a short time, like an hour, to begin with, and slowly increase in duration. In some cases, your first experience might last only a few minutes.

FACTS

Nurse-midwife Susan Luddington introduced kangaroo care to the United States. She had traveled to Bogota, Columbia, and seen it used in hospitals that lacked isolettes for newborns. Skin-to-skin care was their low-tech solution, and the results are remarkable.

With the exception of breastfeeding, a father is just as capable of providing the benefits of kangaroo care as a mom is. It's a good opportunity for your partner to bond with your baby and a good opportunity for you to take a break.

Multiple Births

One of the challenges multiples often have to overcome is premature birth. Low birthweight and other complications of prematurity make it especially important for twins and triplets to get all the health benefits your milk provides. If your babies are confined to NICU or unable to feed at your breast for other medical reasons, they still benefit from your breastmilk. Follow the advice on preemies in the section above and stay confident.

All the regular recommendations given to nursing moms go double (or triple) for mothers of multiples. Get lots of rest, make sure to drink plenty of water, and eat a healthy diet. Feeding more than one baby takes a lot out of you. You've got to take extra care of yourself. Along with lots of time, support, and supplies, you'll need a feeding strategy. Will you nurse them one at a time or together?

One at a Time

If you choose to nurse your infants individually, your partner can keep one entertained while you feed the other. He can sing and cuddle the waiting child or even offer the baby a clean finger to suck on. Once a good nursing routine is established (in about six weeks), your partner can offer one of the babies a bottle of expressed breastmilk. Alternate which baby gets the breast first at each feeding or you might end up with a child who prefers the bottle. Dad can also use alternative methods, like spoon or cup feeding.

Individual feedings give you a wonderful opportunity to spend quality one-on-one time with each of your precious babies. However, while this is a great approach for bonding, some mothers might feel a bit overwhelmed by the almost constant nursing.

Two Breasts, No Waiting

Most mothers of multiples find that feeding both babies at once is an effective way to streamline the nursing process and free up some time for other activities. Multiples are usually comforted by each other's presence, so they might actually prefer to dine together. After all, they shared some pretty crowded living space for those first nine months!

When both babies nurse at once, they'll probably sleep at the same time, too. Remember, when your babies sleep, you sleep, too. If you're not tired enough to nap, take a little personal time. You've earned it.

Tandem Nursing Supplies

Pillows are the single most important breastfeeding accessory when you're nursing two babies at once. Unless you look like Shiva, the Indian goddess with eight arms, you won't be able to hold two babies and manipulate two breasts simultaneously. Pillows elevate both babies to the correct height for nursing and keep them safely in position while leaving your hands free. Usually you'll want a pillow on each side of you. Two more pillows go on your lap. After a while, you'll be able to feed both your babies at once and still have a hand free to hold your glass of water or catch one of your little wiggleworms if he squirms out of position.

Tandem Nursing Positions

The football hold and the crisscross hold are the two most commonly used positions for breastfeeding twins simultaneously. However, any position that works for you is fine. Some women prefer to lie down and lay one baby over their shoulder and the other in an armpit. Experiment until you find a position that you like. Any position you end up using should meet at least the following criteria:

FIGURE 10-1:
Football
(clutch) hold

FIGURE 10-2:
Crisscross
hold

FIGURE 10-3:
Layered hold

It will take flexibility, patience, and practice for you all to work out which method and position works best for you. Pay extra attention to the babies' position, both to ensure that you're not putting additional strain on your neck and back, and to prevent poor (or sliding) latch from hurting your nipples.

Safety—from falling or suffocation

Mobility—lets you keep at least one hand free

Bonding—allows skin-to-skin contact, smell, voice, and (ideally) sight

Positioning—allows proper latch-on and alignment of babies' heads and bodies

Comfort—for everyone involved

Longevity—can be maintained for long periods of time

Triplets

When it's time to breastfeed triplets, you can only feed two at a time. As soon as one finishes, let the third baby nurse. Another option is to give the third infant a bottle of expressed milk while your other two nurse. Put the third infant in his car seat or carrier and rock him until it's his turn. Always rotate which baby waits.

Milk Supply

The key to building and maintaining an adequate milk supply is frequent feedings at the breast. You can easily produce plenty of milk for twins and even triplets. It's simply a matter of supply and demand. If your babies are frequent, eager nursers, your breasts will increase production. You should have no problem producing enough milk if you follow a few basic guidelines.

It's best to avoid using a bottle to feed expressed milk to your infants until they've established a strong nursing routine. Bottle feeding can lead to nipple confusion in newborns. Babies suck differently on bottle nipples than they do on breasts. A baby who gets used to a bottle might breastfeed less effectively, causing your milk production to decrease. If you have to supplement nursing in the first few weeks of life, use a feeding technique that doesn't involve a nipple, such as a spoon or cup.

If you suspect your milk supply is inadequate, evaluate your babies' progress using the information in Chapter 7. The best way to ensure that your babies get what they need is to simply let them nurse often. If frequent nursing doesn't seem to be working, contact a certified lactation consultant immediately.

In order to maintain equal milk production in both breasts, alternate sides between babies at a regular interval. You can rotate every feeding, every day, or anywhere in between. Whatever schedule you decide on should be easy for you to remember.

Some women don't alternate sides. They assign a breast to each baby and nurse only him on that breast. The only effect this is likely to have is that one breast might get larger than the other if one baby is a more vigorous feeder.

If your babies can't adequately stimulate your milk production, use a breast pump. This technique is often utilized when a mother is unable to nurse her child directly because of hospitalization or some other necessary separation. If pumping becomes necessary, you should do it at the times your infants would normally nurse. To increase your milk supply, pump more frequently. It's frequency, not duration, that builds a milk supply.

C-Sections

A Caesarean section delivery necessitates some special attention for breastfeeding. As soon as you know you'll be having a C-section, it's important that you remind your doctor of your desire to breastfeed your baby. Let him or her know that you want to breastfeed immediately following birth. Your doctor and the anesthesiologist will work with you, providing anesthesia and follow-up pain medications that are compatible with lactation.

ESSENTIALS

Although you might want to have your baby room in with you at the hospital, you might find it difficult at first. Some moms manage it, but others need a little extra time to recover from surgery. It's usually best to work your way up to full-time mothering over the first few days postpartum.

A C-section is major surgery and your body needs time to recover. Follow your doctor's instructions. Bed rest is often advised even after you return home. Your baby can stay in the room with you, either next to the bed in a bassinet or alongside you in bed. Keep your supplies within arm's reach and rely on your husband or another helper as much as possible. When you feel up to it, get out of bed and walk around. Movement helps you heal. Just take it slow.

Down's Syndrome

Many babies born with Down's syndrome can nurse without too much difficulty. However, Down's babies do tend to have less muscle tone than other infants, so take special care supporting their heads while they nurse. The football hold allows the most control over your baby's positioning.

Another result of poor muscle tone is an ineffective suck. Suck training can help Down's syndrome infants. To be effective, suck training should be performed two or three times before each feeding. A lactation consultant will teach you effective methods that will work with your infant.

HOW CAN A MOTHER SUCK TRAIN HER BABY?

1. Put your clean finger into his mouth.
2. Hold your finger gently against the roof of his mouth.
3. When baby sucks, slowly turn your finger over.
4. Press down gently on his tongue.
5. Slowly extract your finger.

Occasionally, infants with Down's are unable to effectively breastfeed. In those rare instances, a supplemental device, like a Haberman feeder, is an appropriate solution. Ask your lactation consultant for more information.

Even when your baby is unable to nurse, your breastmilk is still his best food. Your milk provides important brain-building fats that formula lacks. Pump often and rest assured that your efforts will help your child develop to his fullest potential.

Cleft Lip or Cleft Palate

A baby with a cleft lip can usually feed at the breast without much difficulty. If the cleft interferes with his suck, you can cover it with your finger or by pushing a fold of breast tissue into it.

Cleft lips are usually repaired within the first few weeks of life. Some doctors advise against breastfeeding until the lip is healed, but this isn't usually necessary. Many mothers put their babies to breast immediately following surgery. The babies are comforted by nursing and the mother's milk supply is maintained. If you choose not to nurse right away, you should pump your breasts to maintain your milk production.

Cleft palates can present more of a challenge. Babies with cleft palates are often unable to keep the breast in their mouths and might have difficulty compressing the milk sinuses beneath the areola. In addition, they tend to get milk into their ears and sinuses through the hole in their palate.

Common solutions include:

- Use the fingers of the hand supporting your breast to hold your baby's head in place. Your palm supports your breast.
- Keep your baby's head slightly higher than your nipple to prevent milk from flowing into the cleft.
- Change the angle at which your baby takes the breast, especially by aiming the nipple away from the opening in his palate.
- Use a dental appliance to cover the hole in the palate.

More serious cases might require the use of a special feeding device like a soft cup. Your lactation consultant can help make breastfeeding work for you and your cleft-palate baby.

Tongue Tie

In a tongue-tied baby, the frenulum, that thin line of tissue that connects the tongue to the bottom of the mouth, is short and tight. The baby's tongue can't extend past the bottom teeth or effectively compress the milk sinuses when breastfeeding.

FIGURE 10-4:
Tongue tie

Babies with this condition generally grow out of it, but in the meantime, nursing can be uncomfortable for mom and unsatisfying for baby. If tongue tie interferes with breastfeeding, talk to your doctor.

The clipping of the frenulum is very minor oral surgery. This simple office procedure takes just minutes and can even be performed by a dentist. Your baby can be back at your breast immediately and nursing will be much improved, but the benefits go beyond breastfeeding. Tongue tie can also interfere with speech development.

Relactating and Adoptive Moms

If you've breastfed before but had to stop, it is possible to relactate. Amazingly, it's also possible to induce lactation when you've never given birth or even been pregnant. Inducing lactation lets adoptive moms and their babies enjoy the special advantages of a breastfeeding relationship.

You'll need to pump every two to four hours, day and night, if you plan to induce lactation. Your new baby will nurse that often, so you need to "tell" your breasts the schedule. A hospital-grade breast pump with a double pumping attachment is your best bet. Some women start to produce milk within three weeks. Some women will need six weeks or more. If you're relactating, the rule of thumb states that it will take at least the same amount of time to begin lactating as has passed since you weaned. If it's been six weeks since you breastfed, it will probably take six weeks to fully relactate. You'll have more success if you enlist the aid of a certified lactation consultant or a supportive pediatrician.

If you're planning on breastfeeding an adopted baby, remember that most adoptive moms need to supplement their breastmilk with formula. Adoptive breastfeeding is best thought of as a psychological experience, not an exclusively nutritional one. However, there are rare cases where women do manage to produce enough milk for exclusive breastfeeding.

Lactation consultants usually recommend a three-step feeding process for relactating.

1. If possible, breastfeed for a few minutes to encourage the baby to associate the breast with feeding. Provide skin-to-skin contact.
2. Supplement the feeding with a supplemental feeding device that can be used while baby nurses.
3. Pump using a high-quality breast pump.

When the time comes to put your baby to the breast, you again have to be patient. Many older babies are often a little reluctant to nurse from a breast at first. They've been bottle fed and may need time to get accustomed to the breast.

Try not to become discouraged if you have little or no visible milk production while pumping. There's something about a real baby, her smell or the feel of her in your arms, that jump-starts lactation like nothing else. Close your eyes while pumping and think about the baby you're going to be holding soon. Creative visualization can affect your whole body.

If your baby is extremely hungry and you're not yet producing much milk, she might be frustrated. Try feeding her a little expressed milk or formula from a spoon or syringe before you breastfeed, or consider using a supplemental feeding device. Put your baby to breast whenever she wants to nurse, but keep it a pleasant experience for both of you. Remember that any human milk is better than none, and the strength of your relationship with your baby is your primary concern.

CHAPTER 11
Nursing on the Go

There's nothing more convenient than breastfeeding when you're on the road. Nature has provided almost everything your baby needs in one convenient package—you! Whether you and your child are going to the grocery store or hopping on an international flight, breastfeeding can be a simple, safe, and comfortable part of your itinerary.

Nursing in Public

Many women feel comfortable nursing their baby wherever they happen to be. It's every breastfeeding pair's right, and never a cause for shame. Still, some women are understandably uncomfortable with the idea of exposing their breasts in public for any reason. We've grown up in a society that promotes the sexuality of breasts over their functionality, but no one should have to feel embarrassed about feeding her child the way nature intended.

There's really not much to see anyway. Many women use a baby blanket or other material to drape over both baby and breast while baby eats. This can be effective, but it can also draw attention to the whole process, not to mention blocking eye contact with your child. The best way to begin a public nursing session is to simply turn away from view and allow your baby to latch onto the breast. Older nurslings are so adept at the process that you can get them to your breast without much worry about exposing your nipple even if you don't turn around.

If you're shy at first, your mate can help by acting as a barrier, shielding you from view as baby latches on. A father's support of public nursing can be a real blessing for a shy mother. Not only does a woman need her partner's support in general, but people are much less inclined to look at a breastfeeding pair when Dad's around.

Once your baby has latched onto the breast, her head will conceal it from view, allowing you to nurse comfortably without concern. However, if your baby likes to release the breast every once in a while and look around, be ready for a little exposure.

Some older babies like to explore their mother's body while they nurse, their busy little hands pulling at clothing and skin alike. If this describes your child, it's a good idea to keep her hands occupied so she doesn't pull up your shirt and expose your other breast. Hold her hands while she nurses or give her a blanket to cuddle.

By rights, you can breastfeed wherever you happen to be when your child is hungry. With experience, you'll learn which options provide you with enough privacy and comfort to breastfeed successfully.

Babywearing

If you want real freedom to nurse anywhere, consider babywearing. Slings keep your hands free while holding your baby right where you want her. The extra folds of cloth let you cover both your child and your breast, so you can nurse discreetly as you shop, eat in a restaurant, or stand in line at Disney World.

Babywearing has other benefits, too. It keeps your little one warm and secure and promotes a healthy emotional attachment. Carried babies cry less than other babies and gain weight quicker. Parents enjoy a calmer, healthier child and find it easier to care for older siblings when they don't have to use both hands to support a baby. Babywearing is also great exercise.

To begin a breastfeeding session using a sling, position your baby on the breast and use one of your hands to keep your little one in place as you walk. You can start moving as soon as your nursling latches on, but try to keep your pace slow and even.

When to Nurse

If you don't like to nurse in public, timing your trips out of the house can be a great help. Since you can't refuse your hungry baby for long, the best strategy is to make sure she's full before you leave home. If you're going to the grocery store, get everything ready and then wait until your baby's next nursing session. Right after she's done, strap her into the car seat carrier and head out the door. Older children respond well to the same strategy and can even use a pacifier or a cup to extend the time between nursing sessions.

If it does become necessary to breastfeed in public, you'll draw much less attention if you begin at the first signs of hunger. If you delay a

Clothing

The right wardrobe is vital for nursing on the go. A two-piece outfit with a top that can be easily pulled up or unbuttoned from the bottom for easy access is best. Try an oversized T-shirt or sweatshirt. For women who prefer dresses, some manufacturers offer attractive designs with cleverly concealed vertical openings for quick access. A little extra material, like pleats or flaps, provides additional cover once your baby has latched on.

The choice of material and design is important, too. Cotton prints are the most suitable fabrics for breastfeeding mothers. Cotton breathes, so your baby can be comfortable snuggled against it. Printed designs help to camouflage any wet spots from leaking milk.

Where to Nurse

Many breastfeeding-friendly shopping malls, restaurants, and theme parks offer family lounges where you can feed your child in a private and comfortable setting. While these areas are often welcome, you're never required to use any special place for breastfeeding. You have a right to nurse your child wherever you are legally allowed to be. However, many women are a little self-conscious about nursing in public, and, for them, family lounges can be a godsend.

If you're more comfortable nursing privately, here are a few other places to try:

- A corner restaurant booth with your back to the room
- In a parking lot in your car
- A department store fitting room
- The back pew or child nursery at church
- The back row at a matinee
- A quiet aisle at the bookstore or library

feeding until your child is crying, everyone will be looking at you as you struggle to get your screaming baby onto the breast. Watch for hunger cues and find a comfortable spot for feeding as soon as your baby lets you know she's ready.

Supplies

Unlike bottle feeding, breastfeeding doesn't tie you down. When you want to go, there's really nothing that you need to take besides your baby, a car seat, and maybe a spare diaper or two. You won't need to pack bottles, mix formula, or carry as many burp cloths as the mother of a bottle-fed baby.

However, while nature gave you everything you need, there are a few additional items that you might want.

- ❑ Baby sling
- ❑ Comfortable nursing bra
- ❑ Clothing that provides easy, discreet access to your breasts
- ❑ A bottle of water for yourself
- ❑ Diapers
- ❑ Baby wipes
- ❑ Burp cloths
- ❑ Rattle or teething toy (nonchokable)
- ❑ Extra-large resealable (or recyclable) plastic bags for dirty items
- ❑ Extra outfit for baby (and a T-shirt for you)
- ❑ Pacifier for infants older than six weeks
- ❑ Lightweight baby blanket

On long journeys without your baby, you should plan to pack:

- ❑ Manual or battery-operated breast pump
- ❑ Spare batteries and pump parts
- ❑ Storage containers
- ❑ Insulated bag large enough to transport all of your expressed milk

Traveling with infants is complicated enough with car seats, strollers, and diaper bags; it only gets worse when you add jars of baby food to your load. Breastfeeding makes it possible for you to take advantage of your relative freedom within the first six months.

Travel by Car

Road trips with your child can be a breeze. There's something almost magical about the way a moving vehicle lulls a baby to sleep. Many parents will testify to the calming effect of a little drive. There are even devices on the market that claim to simulate the sensation of a running car when hooked onto a baby's crib.

On long road trips, the combination of breastfeeding and riding in the car works to your advantage. If you feed your baby before you begin the drive, you can probably expect her to fall asleep in the car and doze contentedly through the first hour or two of travel. When she wakes up, take a break. Pull into a rest area or any convenient parking lot and feed her. Get out and stretch your legs. Take your baby for a brief stroll, change her diaper, and get ready for the next leg of your journey.

Never remove your child from his car seat for a feeding unless the car is safely parked. All children need to be secured in approved safety restraints whenever the car is on the road. Fussy babies can be calmed with music, toys, or even a clean finger to suck on.

On long rides, babies will often sleep more than they would at home. While that makes for a peaceful drive, all that rest can leave your child up later at night than you'd like. It's a good idea to wake your baby at least every three hours for a feeding. You might even want to keep your baby awake as long as possible as you near your destination.

Another alternative used by parents of young children is to travel by night. With your children sleeping peacefully for long stretches of time, you can cover a lot of distance without interruptions. The car is quiet and the traffic is light.

Travel by Plane

If you're uncomfortable nursing in public, you might be worried about traveling by plane with your baby. However, the high-backed seats of a commercial airliner give you a fairly private setting for nursing. The only people who can see you are the ones seated in the same row as you and anyone who walks past. With that in mind, it's usually best to ask for a window seat near the middle of the plane, with your husband or traveling companion seated next to you. The majority of passenger foot travel is headed toward the bathrooms at the front and back of larger aircraft. When you're seated in the middle, passersby will be kept to a minimum. With your partner blocking your rowmates' view, you can feed your baby in privacy.

FACTS

Most airlines allow you to bring a car seat carrier onboard with you, even if you haven't paid for your child's seat. As long as the flight isn't fully booked, you can use it. Ask a flight attendant to help you move to a pair of empty seats if the flight is open.

If you find yourself in a plane with only one bathroom, try to book a seat as far away from it as possible. If all else fails, ask your flight attendant for assistance. He or she will be glad to get you a blanket to use as a screen, along with extra pillows. There might even be a more private seat open that you can use.

Ideally, you want your baby to be breastfeeding at takeoff and landing. These are the times when the air pressure in the cabin is changing quickly and can cause ears to pop. Sucking and moving the jaws help to equalize the pressure within your baby's ears by way of the eustachian tubes that connect her ears to her mouth. It's the same relief you get by chewing gum.

Depending on your travel time to the airport, your check-in time and boarding delays, it might work to your advantage to feed your baby just before leaving the house. Sometimes, the numbers just don't work out in your favor and you'll find yourself with a hungry baby as you wait in the airport terminal. If she seems hungry, nurse her in the terminal. A deserted passenger gate can be a comfortable and private location. Nurse her again at takeoff. Even if she's not hungry, she'll probably suckle for comfort.

Immunization Recommendations

If you're planning to travel overseas, you might need some immunizations depending on your destination. According to the U.S. Centers for Disease Control, all immunizations currently given to travelers are compatible with breastfeeding. However, the CDC also advises breastfeeding mothers that many of the immunities they acquire through immunization will not necessarily protect their nursing children. It's also not safe to give babies those particular shots directly.

Children are immunized according to a well-established schedule that takes into account their physical development. The CDC recommends that this normal immunization schedule be followed regardless of your travel destination.

The CDC cautions parents of newborns to seriously consider the risk of disease in certain parts of the world. Infants in the first few months of life are especially vulnerable to infectious diseases.

What can you do to protect your child? The CDC advises women with infants or toddlers to breastfeed throughout their trip. Breastfeeding enhances a child's immune system, protecting her from a whole host of infections. As an added benefit, breastfed children aren't exposed to potentially impure local water supplies and foods.

Going Solo

If your work includes a long-distance trip or two where you will be unable to take your baby, you'll have to pack a breast pump. Because your milk production is based on supply and demand, you will need to express your milk regularly while you're away from your child. You can pump and dump, pump and donate your milk to a local milk bank (do the research before you travel), or pump and store.

Freshly pumped breastmilk can be stored safely at room temperature for up to ten hours. Refrigerated breastmilk can be stored for five days. Frozen milk can be stored much longer. If you plan to use your expressed milk, it's best to cool it as soon as possible. Use an insulated soft vinyl lunch bag and ice until you can get to a refrigerator.

Remember to pack extra batteries for handheld pumps, and to purchase appropriate electrical adaptors if you are traveling overseas. Additional spare parts and collection containers can be hard to find when you're across the country, so pack those, too.

ESSENTIALS

If your travels include overseas destinations, you will need to express some milk during the flight for comfort. Again, be sure to bring either a battery-operated pump or a manual model. Most aircraft don't have electricity available to passengers outside of the bathrooms.

In the event that you find yourself away from home without a pump, hand expression is a viable option. However, you probably won't be able to express enough milk to maintain your supply with hand expression alone. If you plan to continue breastfeeding your baby when you return home, you'll need to remove as much milk as possible. Hand expression is really best utilized as a comfort measure to relieve engorgement. Purchase a good pump as soon as possible.

Nursing on the go can be a liberating experience. As more and more states enact laws to protect a breastfeeding mother's right to nurse her child, more women feel empowered to bring breastfeeding back into the public eye. Anywhere it's appropriate to bottle feed, it's appropriate to breastfeed.

CHAPTER 12

Express Yourself

Madonna did it. So did Celine Dion, Cindy Crawford, Anita Baker, Andie McDowell, Demi Moore, Faith Hill, Goldi Hawn, Lisa Kudrow, and Heather Locklear. They were all nursing moms who breastfed and expressed milk for their babies. Whether you're returning to work, relieving engorgement, or pumping milk so you can have a night out, at some point all nursing mothers need to learn the art of expression.

Pump It Up!

A breast pump is not as effective in removing milk from your breasts as your baby is, so it's important to establish a consistent routine to maintain your supply. The more frequently you pump, the stronger your supply will be, the same way frequent nursing works with your baby.

A New Routine

Begin to express your milk about two weeks before returning to work. This will help increase your production and get you into a pumping routine. You'll want to express about the same time as your baby would naturally nurse each day, or about every two to three hours in a twenty-four-hour period.

Begin pumping for fifteen minutes using a double pump, or thirty minutes using a single pump (fifteen minutes on each side).

QUESTIONS?

How can you tell if you are expressing a "normal" amount of milk?
Breasts develop their own general flow pattern. They start dripping, then squirt, then drip, then slow to stop. Continue to pump until the milk stops flowing or dripping.

You might notice that not much milk is expressed the first few times you try. It takes time for your body to get used to this artificial suction device. It also takes time for your milk to letdown. Eventually, you'll notice steady streams and bonafide long-distance sprays from your nipples, but for now, don't worry. Any milk you express is important for your baby's growth. After about a week, you should be able to pump twenty-five ounces or more per day.

When Should I Pump?

Your prolactin levels fluctuate throughout the day. They're lowest in the evening and highest in the morning. If you express your milk in the morning, you will have greater volume. Pump before you wake your baby.

You can still nurse her because your breasts are never really empty. Pump again one and a half to two hours later.

Milk flows best when you're relaxed. If you have difficulty with letdown when you pump, nurse your baby on one breast while pumping the other. Once your baby engages your milk ejection reflex, your milk will flow more freely.

Manual Expression

Sometimes, particularly if you are engorged, your baby might have a difficult time finding enough nipple to take into her mouth. You might need to manually express some milk to relieve the fullness in your breasts and provide some elasticity to your nipple and areola.

Manual expression is the least expensive kind of "pumping." It can be easy with practice, but it can be difficult to learn. If done incorrectly, it can cause bruising, tissue damage, or chafed skin. Ask a lactation consultant or health care provider to demonstrate the correct technique. Seeing it in action is different than reading about it in a book. Practice manual expression even if you don't intend to make it a daily routine. At some point you might need to express your milk without the use of a pump.

FIGURE 12-1: Breast massage

FIGURE 12-2: Manual expression

Eventually, you can try the two-handed, doubled-breasted method while sitting at a table and expressing milk into a large pan. If you don't intend to store your milk for later, you can also express your milk in a warm shower.

THE HOW-TO'S OF MANUAL EXPRESSION

1. Wash your hands and gather a clean collection container. A wide-mouth cup strategically placed in front of the nipple will catch your milk as it squirts. Some mothers place a funnel inside a baby bottle to collect their milk.

2. Gently massage your breasts. Use small circular motions as if you're conducting a breast self-exam, or you can do whatever feels comfortable. Start on the outside of the breast and move toward the areola. Bend over at the waist and let gravity assist you. The key is to relax and allow letdown to occur. Warm washcloths applied to the breast will also help.

3. Place your thumb and first two fingers about one inch behind the nipple or on the edge of the areola in a twelve o'clock and six o'clock position. Your fingers will resemble the letter C.

4. Lift your breast and push it back toward your ribcage.

5. Press down toward the nipple in a gently rolling motion to compress milk out of the sinuses, the way your baby does when she nurses. Don't squeeze the nipple, just the sinuses under the areola. Release your hold and do this again.

6. When milk begins to slow, rotate your hand position around the breast (i.e., eleven and five o'clock) and continue until the sinuses are empty. Work all sides of the breast until milk no longer flows or drips.

7. Rub excess milk onto your nipple and areola.

Breast Pump Selection

If you intend to express your milk on a regular basis, you'll want to choose a breast pump that meets your individual needs. Criteria vary from person to person, and even over time for the individual. Keep your ultimate goal (whatever it may be) in mind while you shop, and consult your doctor or lactation consultant.

How often will you use a pump: daily, weekly, or as needed? Are you returning to work or just planning to express an occasional bottle for date night?

What can you afford? Is this an investment that you intend to use again with other babies or would it be more economical for you to rent?

Will you be transporting your breast pump to work? Will you need a cooler or carrying case to transport milk back home?

Will you be expressing in your car?

What are your power sources?

How much time do you have to express your milk?

What kinds of accessories will you need?

When choosing a pump, select the one that most closely imitates your baby's suckling pattern. Pumps that offer the most cycling per minute are the best. Look for pumps that offer thirty-four to fifty cycles per minute. That timing is most like your baby's nursing pattern. You also want a pump with adjustable suction rates.

QUESTIONS?

Where can I find more information about breast pump rentals?
The companies listed below are leaders in breast pump rentals, and their pumps are carried by most hospitals and maternal/child health organizations.

In the selection of a breast pump, you truly get what you pay for. Better pumps will cost more, but they express more milk in a shorter period of time, are more comfortable to use, and are less likely to cause tissue damage.

Contact a lactation consultant or certified breastfeeding educator about the different pumps available. They'll share the pros and cons of each model with you and can give you additional information about where to purchase or rent a quality pump. You can also call or go to the Web sites of the following companies:

Hollister/Ameda/Egnell	800-323-4060	*www.Hollister.com*
Medela	800-835-5968	*www.Medela.com*
White River	800-824-6351	*www.whiteriver.com*

You can also contact your local WIC office, a lactation consultant or breastfeeding educator, or your local birthing center for additional information and recommendations.

Types of Breast Pumps

It's important to choose a reputable brand like Medela or Hollister. These manufacturers have years of experience and a solid history behind their products. A breast pump is an important tool, not a toy. You wouldn't go to a seafood place if you wanted steak, so don't buy a breast pump from a company that specializes in something else.

Check out breast pumps in consumer product safety reports. It's a handy way to compare products based on durability, repair frequency, cost, and any other criteria that are important to you. It's also the place to find out about safety notices and recalls.

Bicycle Horn Pump

Shaped like a bicycle horn, these pumps are the least expensive, but they're also the least effective. You create suction by squeezing and releasing the bulb. Milk is collected into the bulb or a depression in the bottom of the horn. However, because the bulbs can't always be disassembled and cleaned, they can become contaminated with bacterial growth. In addition, bicycle horn pumps can cause breast tissue damage. Unless you are pumping and dumping, this is one to avoid.

Hand- or Foot-Operated Pumps

There are several hand pumps on the market and making a decision about the right one is a difficult task. Most hand pumps offer cylinder-style action or handgrip operation. With cylinder pumps you pull on a piston or plunger to create suction. The flange (a funnel-like contraption) is centered over your nipple. You push the plunger in, then pull it out to draw milk from the breast sinuses.

Handgrip pumps work in much the same way. They provide suction through the squeeze of a bar. These offer convenient one-handed operation.

Foot-pedal pumps are basically manual pumps that you work with your feet. A hose runs from the pedal to the flange. Foot pedal pumps offer double pumping, which is the most effective method of expression.

Each of the manual breast pumps is effective and offers good exercise, but they might wear you out. They are best for occasional use only.

Handheld Battery-Operated Pumps

Battery-operated pumps use a small motor to produce suction. Older pumps require you to manually release the suction, while newer models offer automatic or button suction-release. The motor creates a vacuum on your nipple/areola and you break suction to create the pseudo-nursing effect. Some pumps offer an automatic release that cycles around four to eight times per minute.

Although handheld battery-operated pumps are affordable, they are not very efficient and can cause tissue damage. They're generally slower to create and release suction, so their action doesn't mimic your baby's suckling. In fact, they're often responsible for a diminished milk supply. Many of these pumps are poorly constructed and seem to break just before their ninety-day warranty expires. In addition, they can be noisy and require frequent battery replacement. They are best used for occasional pumping only.

Portable Electric Pumps

These pumps are durable and easy to transport, but often don't offer the optimum number of suction-release cycles. Like many handheld battery-operated machines, some electric pumps depend on the user to break suction. Portable electric pumps often come with accessory packages that offer cigarette lighter adaptors for use in your automobile. They are more effective if you have an abundant milk supply. They also have adjustable suction rates.

Hospital-Grade Pumps

These are simply the best and most efficient pumps around. Although they can be expensive to purchase, most hospitals offer rental options for women who intend to pump frequently. Hospital-grade pumps come in several sizes and weights. Some are as light as four pounds while others weigh up to twenty pounds. The lightweight pumps are easily transported and come with adaptors for automobile use.

FIGURE 12-4: Hospital-grade pump

Look for a pump that provides an automatic suction-release cycle that mimics your baby's suck. Most cycle around forty-eight to sixty times per minute. These pumps offer double pumping, are great for establishing a strong milk supply, and are perfect for the working mother or for use when you have a hospitalized infant. Sometimes hospital-grade pumps are covered by insurance, particularly if your baby is premature or has a medical condition. Suzanne's doctor simply wrote a letter to the insurance company about the benefits of breastfeeding a low-birthweight infant, and they covered all pump expenses for six months. Hospital-grade pumps are the most effective as well as cost-efficient—if you use them on a daily basis. Rental fees for these pumps range from one to three dollars per day.

Pump Process (Twenty to Thirty Minutes)

1. Wash your hands with soap and water.
2. Wash all breast pump equipment and assemble it according to the manufacturer's directions.
3. Find a comfortable location to express, just as you would to nurse your baby.
4. Gently massage your breasts or apply a warm washcloth.
5. Center the nipple in the plastic flange. If you are using an electric or battery-operated pump, turn it on the lowest/slowest setting first and increase the speed to match your baby's suck. If you are using a cylinder pump, pull the piston away from your breast, push it back in, and pull it out again. Try to mimic one suck per second.

Watch how your nipple enters and exits the flange. If your nipple is squashed, you might need a larger flange neck. Nipples should not rub or touch the sides. Contact the vendor you purchased your kit from to see about their return policy.

6a. Pump the first breast for about seven minutes. (If you are using a double pump, note that you'll follow the pump-massage-pump procedure without switching breasts.)
6b. Switch sides and pump the second breast for seven minutes.
7. Massage your breasts a second time.
8. Return to the first breast for five to seven minutes or until milk no longer flows, followed by the second breast for the same amount of time.
   Note: You might have to exchange containers midway through your expression session if your collection bottle becomes full.
9. When milk stops dripping, release suction at the breast as you would with your infant.
10. When you're finished, rub any excess milk onto your nipples and areola.
11. Pour the milk into a clean container for storage, or, if a lid is provided with your pump, screw it on tightly.

12. Label your milk with the date and the amount, and immediately refrigerate what you don't plan to use within eight to ten hours.
13. Detach the pump and disassemble any washable components. Clean everything according to the instructions in hot, soapy water. Air dry the components on a paper towel or a clean dishcloth.

Storage of Human Milk

After you've expressed your breastmilk, you will need to store it if it's not immediately given to your baby. Human milk can be stored at room temperature, refrigerated, or frozen. Each requires different handling and storage procedures. Temperature is the single most important factor in determining the length of time it's safe to store your milk.

STORAGE TIME GUIDELINES	
Room Temperature	6–10 hours
Refrigerator	5–8 days
Freezer Inside a Refrigerator	2 weeks
Self-Defrosting Freezer w/Separate Door	3–6 months
Deep Freeze at 0 degrees	6–12 months

Defrosted or thawed milk can be stored for up to twenty-four hours in the refrigerator. If you don't have a refrigerator at your work site, you can refrigerate milk in an insulated cooler with ice packs until you get home or to the day care.

Store your cooled or frozen milk in the back of your refrigerator. It's cooler there and your milk will be less affected by temperature changes from the frequent opening and closing of the door.

Studies have found that the antibacterial properties of breastmilk actually protect it from bacterial growth while it's stored in a bottle. That's why human milk can be stored at room temperature for up to ten hours. However, if you don't intend to use your milk for some time, it's best refrigerated. Discard any unused portion left in the bottle after your baby has eaten. It's hard to watch that liquid gold go down the drain, but bacteria from your baby's mouth make it unsafe for future feedings.

Critically ill infants require different breastmilk handling and storage techniques than full-term, healthy infants. The hospital lactation consultant or NICU staff will work closely with you on expression and storage.

Plastic versus Glass Debate

Every couple of years breastfeeding educators learn about new studies that change the recommended practice for storing human milk. A few years ago, plastic was the container of choice. Then there was a concern about chemicals in plastic that might leach into milk. As a result, glass was recommended. Soon afterward, studies indicated that lycocytes, or living cells, clung to the sides of glass bottles. That made researchers question whether infants were actually receiving all of the benefits of breastmilk. Today, new plastics have been developed in response to chemical leakage concerns and best practice is back to plastic.

For many years, women have been freezing breastmilk in both metal and hard plastic ice cube trays. Once frozen, the cubes are removed and stored in freezer bags. Current research indicates no harm or benefit to this practice.

Plastic—If you're freezing breastmilk in plastic bottles or liner bags, leave at least an inch at the top. As liquids freeze, they expand. Mark the date and amount on the outside of the bottle or bag. You can use wax pencils or masking tape. Be sure to add your baby's name if the bottle will be used at a day care center. If you're freezing breastmilk in a bottle liner, double bag your milk to decrease the chances of seam leakage. If you have an extra bottle handy, freeze milk with bags still in the bottle to preserve their shape. Bottle liners that are intended for the long-term storage of human milk are the best.

Freeze milk in amounts of two to four ounces. That way, it will thaw more quickly and less will go to waste. When baby consistently takes eight ounces at a single feeding, you can safely freeze your milk in larger amounts, but larger amounts take longer to thaw.

Glass—Glass bottles have long been the storage container of choice for lactation consultants and breastfeeding educators. Because milk expands when frozen, be careful to leave adequate space available in the bottle for this process. Glass bottles can break if you fill them all the way to the top. Again, freeze in smaller amounts.

Ice Cube Trays—Metal ice cube trays can be purchased at gourmet food stores. Simply pour liquid into the tray and seal the whole thing inside a large freezer bag, or cover it tightly with plastic wrap or aluminum foil. Pop out the cubes as needed. If the cubes are too large to fit into the mouth of the bottle, thaw them inside the refrigerator in another container and transfer the milk to a bottle when it's ready.

Containers should be clean, but they don't need to be sterilized. If you have a sick or hospitalized infant, talk to a lactation consultant or NICU personnel. Wash containers and all pumping equipment in hot, soapy water and let them air dry on a paper towel or clean dishcloth. You don't need to wash tubes or other components of the breast pump if they haven't come in contact with your milk.

Thawing Frozen Breastmilk

The recommendation for thawing breastmilk is to let it stand in the refrigerator overnight. Milk will thaw slowly and consistently over a twelve-hour period, and faster if frozen in smaller amounts.

Do not refreeze thawed milk or reheat heated milk. Throw away any milk remaining in your baby's bottle and always use the oldest milk first.

Another common method of thawing milk is to place a bottle of frozen milk in a pan of warm water and change the water frequently to replace any lost heat. You can also run bottled milk under a warm running faucet.

Breastmilk separates into milk and fat (cream). The fat floats to the top. Once your breastmilk is thawed, gently shake or swirl the bottle to mix it all up again. Thawed milk sometimes smells "soapy," but that doesn't mean it's sour or has gone bad. It usually happens in response to defrosting the fat in the milk.

Heating Fresh Milk

Your breastmilk is the perfect temperature for your baby. Even when it's been stored at room temperature, fresh milk doesn't need to be heated. Boiling causes the milk to lose its precious immunity-enhancing properties. Even a slight warm-up in the microwave can hurt the milk and possibly harm your baby. Microwave heat is uneven and causes hot spots in a bottle that will scald baby's mouth. If you decide to refrigerate your milk, you can heat it by holding the bottle under warm tap water or letting it stand in a bowl or pan of warm water.

It's best to use your breastmilk in the first few days after you've expressed it. Breastmilk is filled with living cells and delicate ingredients that are meant for your child immediately. Breastmilk loses many of its disease-fighting properties with freezing, with boiling, and over time. Although it's still the most perfect nutrition for your child, the near magical immunity properties of your milk are important, too!

Pump Up the Volume!

Your milk supply will decrease the first week you return to work. If that return happens at six weeks postpartum, your baby also hits a growth spurt at this time. Remember to express milk often on a regular schedule to keep up with your baby's demands. Nurse as soon as you greet your infant, even if it's in your child care provider's home. Your milk supply will catch up within a few days.

What about Dads?

Have Dad set up the pump and keep you supplied with warm washcloths. If you prefer to pump in privacy, make it your partner's special time with your new baby. Dad can help out by making your pumping experience as relaxing as possible. Anything that helps you relax also helps you to letdown your milk. A good foot-rub while you pump can be wonderful. So can a shoulder massage. If he can control himself, teach him the fine art of breast massage.

If you've begun to offer your baby an occasional bottle of expressed milk, this is the perfect time for your partner to participate in the feeding of your baby. A bottle of expressed milk in the refrigerator means that anyone can handle those midnight feedings. Let the games begin . . .

CHAPTER 13

Bottle Feeding
Your Baby

If you've been nursing your baby at all, way to go! You've given your baby a loving, healthy start. If you're going to bottle feed now, you need to make a few informed decisions. Are you going to continue with breastmilk or switch to formula, or use both? If you choose to add formula to your routine, how does that work? And then there are bottles and nipples to consider.

Bottles, Nipples, and Other Supplies

Whether you are incorporating formula into your routine, or need bottles for expressed milk, your considerations will be the same: comfort and safety for your child, and simplicity for you. Remember that your child is used to your breast, so it's important to find a product that he can adjust to easily.

Bottles

Whether you choose to use plastic or glass bottles is up to you. Glass is the preferred material for breastmilk, but either is fine for formula. Bottles come in two basic styles: liner bottles and traditional.

Liner bottles use disposable sterile bags. The liner fits on the inside of a bottomless tube "bottle." Once you screw the nipple on the top and squeeze any extra air out of the bottle liner, you have a bottle baby can drink from in any position. Your baby is also less likely to suck air, which can cause spitting up or tummy aches.

FACTS

If your baby has been breastfed exclusively for at least twelve months, you can skip this section. Babies that age don't need a bottle and should be ready to go straight to a cup or straw. If you introduced the cup at six months, she's probably an old pro by now. It's easier to wean a baby just once!

Other bottles look like the traditional baby bottle we all recognize. The milk or formula goes into the bottle directly. The nipple and ring (or one-piece nipple-ring) screw onto the top. You don't need to buy bottle liners, but you do need to keep the bottle tilted enough to fill the nipple with formula. Otherwise, baby might swallow some air.

There are quite a few new twists on the old-style, traditional bottle. Angled bottles have a sharp bend toward the nipple end. That makes it easier to keep the nipple full by allowing you to hold the bottle up without making baby strain after the nipple. There are also bottles shaped like an elongated O, with a hole in the middle. These are easier for a baby's tiny hand to grasp.

Nipples

The single most important thing to consider when choosing a nipple is the flow speed. A nipple that lets too much formula out too fast can choke your newborn or let her take in too much air. A low-flow nipple is perfect for newborns. However, your older child may grow frustrated if she has to work too hard at sucking. Check packaging labels for the flow rate when purchasing new nipples.

Once you've selected the proper flow rate for your baby, it's time to let your baby make some choices. Every baby has a preference for one type of bottle nipple over the others. Playtex Nursernipples, standard bottle nipples, latex, rubber, or silicone—your baby might be willing to use several of these but will probably prefer one or two. If baby uses her tongue to eject the nipple before she's fed or otherwise refuses the bottle, try another style. When you find what she likes, stick with it. Having said that, here's a quick look at the different nipples available.

Wide-Based—Most Playtex liner-style bottles use either a rounded or squared-off, wide-based, soft nipple. If you thought breastfed babies sucked only on Mom's nipples, you'd probably think Playtex was the most naturally shaped bottle nipple. It's not. However, if you're exclusively bottle feeding, that's no big deal. If you prefer a more natural shape but like the Playtex disposable bottle system, you're in luck. Playtex makes orthodontic nipples, too.

Orthodontic—Orthodontic nipples are shaped to resemble what a mother's nipple and areola look like inside a nursing baby's mouth. They are longer and flatter than standard bottle nipples. They come in two sizes. Number 1 is small and designed for premature infants and smaller newborns. Number 2 is fine for most other babies. Orthodontic nipples are called orthodontic because they might help your child's mouth and jaws grow more naturally, as if she were breastfed. Bear in mind that the whole nipple goes into the baby's mouth, not just the tip. There is also a top and bottom to some orthodontic nipples. If you put them into baby's mouth upside down, not much formula can get out. Although orthodontic nipples might be more like real breastfeeding, some babies gag and refuse to use them.

Standard—Standard bottle nipples are inexpensive, easy-to-find, and can work as well as any other style when properly used. Lately, there's been an explosion in the variety of these "old-fashioned" nipples. You can buy them made from a variety of materials, angled, or with air-excluding valve systems.

FIGURE 13-1:
Wide-Based

FIGURE 4-2:
Orthodontic

FIGURE 13-3:
Standard

For many years, bottle nipples were manufactured from rubber. Today, silicone has become the material of choice for many parents. Silicone lasts longer than rubber or latex. Unlike traditional materials, silicone has no taste or odor. It's also transparent, so you can see how much milk is in the nipple and be confident that the nipple is clean.

Make it a habit to check nipples for wear and deterioration at every cleaning. Grasp the nipple between your thumb and forefinger. Hold the base with your other hand and pull. The nipple should snap back firmly. Immediately replace any torn, sticky, swollen, or cracked bottle nipples.

Pacifiers

All babies need to suck. Even if she isn't hungry, sucking can calm and comfort a fussy baby. Breastfeeding moms are advised against the use of pacifiers until a solid nursing routine is established, but bottle-fed babies can use them immediately. Try to stick with the same nipple design as your baby's bottle.

Pacifiers are made in one of two ways. One-piece construction means the entire pacifier is molded at once from the same material. Composite construction means that the nipple is attached to separately molded parts made from different materials. The one-piece style is the safest. They're a little harder to find, but the extra peace of mind is worth the effort.

PACIFIER SAFETY CHECKLIST:

❑ One-piece construction
❑ No attached cord or strings, clips, or decorations
❑ Vent holes in the shield
❑ Large and firm enough that it cannot bend or fit into baby's mouth

The U.S. Consumer Products Safety Commission lists pacifier recalls on its Web site back to 1984. Of the twenty-one recalls, at least seventeen were for composite pacifiers. The most common problem was small parts that presented a choking hazard. Just like bottle nipples, pacifier nipples wear out and become unsafe. Check them after every washing.

Keeping It Clean

Bottles and nipples should be as clean as possible. If you normally wash dishes with unchlorinated water, or if your baby is a preemie or has weakened immunity, everything needs to be boiled. Bring a pan of water to a full, rolling boil and drop in nipples, bottles, and other utensils that come in contact with your child's food. Let these items boil for five minutes. After everything's cooled, wash your hands well with soap and prepare the bottles.

ESSENTIALS As you would with any canned food, wipe the top of the formula can off with a clean cloth before opening. You can be confident that the contents of the can are sanitary, but you don't know what's been on the outside.

If you live in a city with chlorinated water, you need to boil only new nipples, once, to remove any chemicals left over from the manufacturing process. After the first use, you can wash them in the sink or top rack of the dishwasher. Repeated boilings can lead to a premature deterioration of the material. Read the instructions that come with your bottle nipples. Some manufacturers don't recommend nipples be washed in the dishwasher at all. Be sure to remove any old formula that might clog the hole in the nipple. Those little holes can plug easily, so force some soapy water through them until they squirt freely. Rinse everything with hot water.

Water

It's important to remember that the formula you choose is only part of what your baby will be consuming. The other part is water. Safe water is vital for babies using formula.

How can you be sure your water is safe enough? As a rule, if your city's water supply meets federal and state guidelines for safety, it should be fine for use in formula preparation. However, there are exceptions, so have your water tested if you live in rural areas or have had seasonal thaws or floods.

Many new parents choose bottled water for their babies' formula, but don't be fooled into assuming it's better than the water coming out of your tap at home. The federal regulations for bottled water are far less stringent than the regulations for your city's tap water. But what about those bottled waters that feature a picture of a happy baby? The name and label don't mean much. Ninety-eight-cents-per-quart "baby water" is not necessarily any better than sixty-seven-cents-per-gallon "drinking water" or less-than-one-cent-per-gallon tap water. The water industry's standards for "baby water" are no better than ordinary city water.

FACTS

If you live in an older house, let the water run for a minute before you use it to remove any lead or impurities that accumulated in the water as it sat in the pipes. Avoid using hot water from the tap. Lead and minerals leach into hot water more easily than into cold. Bacteria prefer warm water, too.

A water filter is another option. A simple pitcher purifier can be purchased cheaply and can hold enough water for a day's worth of formula. You can also install water-filtering systems on your taps or on the water supply to your entire house. If you choose to filter your water at home, remember to change your filter cartridges regularly. Old filter cartridges can be an ideal breeding ground for germs.

Formula

Premanufactured infant formula is a recent invention. Chemist and merchant Henri Nestle claimed to produce the first commercially available artificial infant food back in 1867. The Nestle Company is still producing infant food today, under the name Carnation. They are one of what we'll refer to as the "Big Three" infant formula manufacturers.

Carnation makes Good Start brand formulas. Ross Laboratories makes Similac. Mead Johnson makes Enfamil. However, these are not the only baby formulas around. Wyeth Nutritionals manufactures infant formulas sold under store brand names throughout the country. At the time of this writing, Wyeth manufactured the following brands:

- Albertson's Baby Basics
- CVS
- HEB
- Kmart
- Kroger

- Meijer
- Target

Store brands of infant formula can be a great way to save money. Wyeth's Web site reports savings of 18 to 42 percent over the three national brands. All infant formula has to be approved by the Food and Drug Administration (FDA), so you know it's safe.

Choosing a Formula

Before you feed your newborn anything besides breastmilk, talk to your doctor. There are many different types and brands of infant formula. Although all of it has to be approved by the FDA as safe and nutritious for babies, there are differences to consider based on your baby's individual needs.

Cows' Milk-Based Formula

This is the meat and potatoes of formulas. It's standard fare for most formula-fed babies from birth to their first birthday. Vitamins, minerals, fats, and sugars are mixed together in a base of cows' milk proteins. If your baby is normal birthweight and healthy, and if you have no reason to suspect food allergies, a regular formula based on modified cows' milk is usually the right choice.

Soy-Based Formula

If your baby is extremely fussy, gassy, or spits up often, talk to your doctor about the possibility of food allergies or a sensitivity to cows' milk protein. If your doctor thinks cows' milk sensitivity is the problem, she'll probably tell you to switch to a soy-based formula. If you're a vegan vegetarian or need to keep kosher, a soy-based formula is the next best thing to breastmilk.

Preemie Formula

Premature babies need formula with a few extras—extra calories, extra proteins, and extra vitamins and minerals. Preemie formulas provide these extras while building on a foundation of milk-based formula. Use of a preemie formula typically begins in the hospital and continues until your doctor recommends a change. Often, babies will switch to a regular formula once they have caught up with other babies their age in terms of size, weight, and energy.

Predigested Formula

The proteins in predigested formula have been broken down so baby can more easily use them. These formulas are useful for colicky babies or others who might have a sensitivity to milk proteins. Although milk-based, these formulas are specially modified to meet the nutritional needs of special babies. Enfamil Pregestimil goes an extra step and provides 55 percent of its fat content in an easier-to-digest form, too. All the predigested formulas are easier on baby's tummy than regular formula. Baby's less fussy, so Mom and Dad are happier, and the formula company's happier because this stuff costs a mint.

Low-Iron Formula

Low-iron formula has less than the recommended daily allowance of iron for your baby. The AAP does not recommend low-iron formula for infants younger than six months of age. Once upon a time, iron was thought to cause constipation in infants, but that's no longer the case. Anemia (low levels of iron in the blood) is the real health threat for growing babies. Use iron-fortified formula until your baby is old enough to get iron from other sources.

Thickened Formula

Thickened formula is recommended only as a last resort for special needs infants. Never use it without a doctor's recommendation. The thickening agent is a modified rice starch. Although approved for babies from birth to twelve months, cereal products like rice starch ordinarily have no place in an infant's diet before four to six months of age. Their little digestive systems are just not up to it. Thickened formulas can be difficult to mix and they sometimes cause large, smelly stools. On the other hand, thickened formulas can be a lifesaver to certain special needs babies who have trouble keeping formula down. Babies with uncomplicated GER are the most likely candidates for a thickened formula.

Follow-Up Formulas

After your baby celebrates her first birthday, she's ready to move beyond formula. Along with all of the wonderful new foods your baby's been trying since she was six months old, your baby can now drink milk—plain, ordinary homogenized whole milk. Follow-up formulas are marketed to parents who are worried about their baby's nutrition. Some follow-ups are marketed to parents of children as young as four months. There is really no reason to switch from a regular formula at such a young age. If your little one is getting proper nutrition in her diet after her first birthday, follow-up formulas are an unnecessary expense.

Powdered, Concentrated, or Ready-to-Feed?

For economy, availability, and shelf life, choose powdered formula mix. Powdered is the old reliable form of infant formula. It's great for around the house. Every store seems to carry it and the price is right. Sure, the difference in cost is only a few cents per feeding, but over the course of a month, that can add up to enough cash for, oh, maybe . . . a baby-sitter? On the down side, formula powder is a little bit messy, preparation is the most complicated (but still pretty simple), and you need safe water.

Concentrated liquid is a nice middle ground between the indulgence of ready-to-feed and the thriftiness of powder. Concentrate is nearly as available as powder. Mixing is simple. The cost is right in between the other two types of formula, too. Concentrated liquid, though, doesn't work well out of the house. Open cans need to be refrigerated immediately, and you've got to have safe water for mixing.

Ready-to-feed is the Rolls Royce of formulas. You can buy it in quart containers or even individual serving bottles with disposable nipples. Sound expensive? It is. Ready-to-feed formula, used exclusively, can easily cost you a dollar per day more than powder. The disposable nipples seem a little wasteful, too, but don't try to reuse them. It's not safe. They are not made for multiple uses. Ready-to-feed formula is unmatched among formulas for traveling convenience. Pack a bunch of single-serving bottles in the diaper bag and you're set for anything.

Feeding with a Bottle

First, get comfortable. Find a place where you can easily support the baby for a length of time without straining yourself. A comfortable chair is a good choice.

Second, tilt the bottle so the nipple is full of formula. Otherwise your baby will swallow excessive amounts of air during feeding. More air equals more spitup.

Third, tilt your baby so that her head is higher than her stomach. Never feed your baby when she is lying down. She can get ear infections. The eustachian tubes connect your baby's mouth and inner ear. When she drinks lying back, fluids run into her inner ear and stay there. Any food warmed to body temperature is like a fertility clinic for bacteria. Sitting up or reclining slightly are the correct positions for feeding.

FACTS

When your baby's first tooth arrives, it's time to begin practicing a good dental routine. Buy a soft, child-sized toothbrush or use a wet cloth. You don't need toothpaste at this age. Make a game of cleaning that precious little tooth. Remember, the goal is to take care of the teeth while getting your child into the habit of good dental hygiene.

Fourth, cuddle your baby. Hold her as if you were breastfeeding. This is especially true for newborns. A newborn's eyes can't focus well beyond about a foot or so. That just happens to be the distance between your eyes and hers when she is breastfeeding. Your baby wants to see you. She wants to interact with you and get to know you. Cuddle your baby while she eats. Coo to her. Sing to her. Take off your shirt and go skin to skin. These activities bring security and comfort to your baby and help you to bond. Sometimes it might seem like you've been feeding her forever, but you'll look back on those early feedings fondly when your little baby isn't so little anymore.

As your baby becomes able to grasp the bottle and take control, let her. Her coordination might be lacking at first. Sometimes babies frustrate themselves by knocking the bottle out of their own mouths. At those times, hold the bottle but let her grasp and tug it around. Before long, she'll be an old pro.

Dad's Turn

Dads and older siblings have a wonderful opportunity to hold and cuddle their babies during bottle feeding. Take turns with the baby or feed in shifts. You're a family now. Make raising your baby a family affair. If you can all be involved, your baby will thrive. Whether you're using formula or breastmilk, your bottle-feeding experience can be very satisfying.

CHAPTER 14

Nutrition for Mom

Breastfeeding moms have nutritional needs above and beyond those of other women. Your milk quality won't usually suffer from poor eating habits, but your own health might. Your body will provide your baby with all the nutrients she needs, even if it means taking them from itself. Many women don't eat a well-balanced diet, so their bodies rob themselves of important nutrients in order to supply their growing infants' needs.

A Healthy Example

When your toddler sees you enjoying good food, she's more likely to enjoy it herself. If you don't like a particular vegetable, she'll pick up on that, too. Getting your child started with a healthy lifestyle is the loving thing to do, and it can be as simple as having healthy food around the house instead of chips and candy.

Fathers can help, too. It's hard to maintain healthy eating habits if your mate isn't following the game plan. Dads should try to stick with a healthy menu around their wives and children whenever possible. It's all too easy to let either parent's bad habit become the family's bad habit. An occasional treat is fine, but if you feel the need to indulge in junk food, practice moderation.

A Word about Water

During lactation, your body uses tremendous amounts of water. While mild dehydration on your part won't affect your milk production in any significant way, it will cause problems for your own overall health. Irritability and a loss of energy and focus are some common symptoms of dehydration.

Moments after sitting down to breastfeed, you'll begin to feel thirsty. Almost every woman does. Get in the habit of taking a glass of water with you every time you nurse. When your baby takes the fluid out, you put it right back in.

Water is the recommended beverage. Juice and soft drinks are too sugary and don't replace your body's fluids as well as water does. A glass or two of fruit juice per day is a healthy addition to your diet, but drinking juice instead of water can lead to unwanted weight gain.

Don't wait until you're thirsty to have a glass of water. Thirst is a late indicator of dehydration. Usually, by the time you feel thirsty, your body is already too dry. If your urine is consistently dark, your mouth is dry, and you suffer from constipation, you're probably dehydrated. Stay ahead of dehydration by drinking eight to ten glasses of water every day, but don't overdo it. Extra water won't increase your milk production.

Food Pyramid

The U.S. Food and Drug Administration publishes the Food Guide Pyramid that we all learned about back in elementary school. It's a handy way to put together a healthy daily menu. The pyramid is built from six food groups.

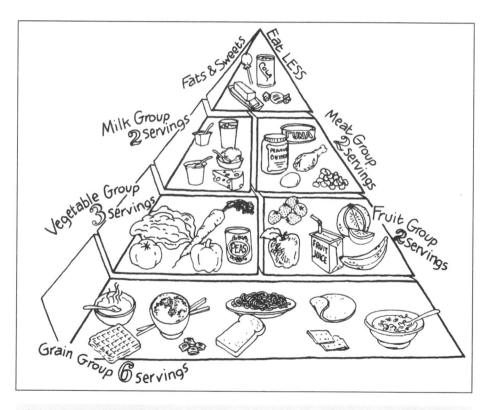

Figure 14-1: Food Pyramid. The FDA does ongoing research on nutrition and provides the public with tools to ensure its heathy eating habits. Use the Food Pyramid as a guide for yourself, and speak with your pediatrician about a similar guide for your child.

Group 1: Bread, Cereal, Rice, and Pasta

The grains group is the base of the Food Pyramid, and foods from this group should make up the majority of your daily diet. Six to eleven servings per day are recommended for breastfeeding women. A serving from this group would be a single slice of bread, one ounce of ready-to-eat cereal, or one-half cup of rice, pasta, or cooked cereal.

Group 2: Vegetable

The vegetable group is a rich source of nutrients but is often neglected in many Americans' diets. Eating three to five servings of vegetables per day is a good start. A serving equals one cup of raw, leafy veggies; one-half cup of cooked or chopped raw vegetables; or three-quarters of a cup of vegetable juice.

Group 3: Fruit

Fruits are delicious and nutritious. Just two to four servings per day will keep you in good shape and give your body the natural sugars it craves. A medium-sized whole fruit; a half-cup of chopped, cooked, or canned fruit; or three-quarters of a cup of fruit juice each count as one serving.

Group 4: Milk, Yogurt, and Cheese

The dairy group is a great source of calcium and is often fortified with vitamin D. WIC recommends four daily servings for women who nurse their babies. One cup of milk or yogurt, one and one half ounces of natural cheese, or two ounces of processed cheese count as a single serving. It's not necessary to drink lots of extra milk when lactating. You don't need milk in your diet to make milk in your breasts.

Group 5: Meat, Poultry, Fish, Eggs, Nuts, and Dry Beans

Incorporate three daily servings from this group, which helps provide essential fats, proteins, vitamins, and minerals in a relatively small package. Consider a serving to consist of two to three ounces of cooked lean meat, two eggs, four tablespoons of peanut butter, or two thirds of a cup of nuts.

Group 6: Fats, Oils, and Sweets

There is no recommended daily intake of foods from group six (sigh!). Use fats, oils, and sweets sparingly. Fats and sugars are important to your health, but most Americans consume too much of them. All the necessary fat and sugar you need is present in the foods from the other five Food Guide groups in healthier amounts and in combination with other nutrients.

While reviewing "Nutrition Facts" on food packaging, be aware that the suggested serving sizes listed reflect the amount of food that the producer considers to be one serving. The serving size recommended by the Food Guide Pyramid is based on the amount of the food necessary for your nutritional needs.

Vitamin and Mineral Supplements

The best way to fulfill all your nutritional requirements is by eating a varied diet from the lower five groups of the Food Pyramid. Whole foods are complex powerhouses of good things for your body. A vitamin C pill might provide all of your required vitamin C, but an orange provides the same benefit as a pill along with fiber, carotene, calcium, simple sugars, and more. Many of the components of whole foods might help us in ways that haven't been discovered yet. We just don't know all there is to know about nutrition. Without a complete knowledge of our nutritional needs, we can't presume to fill those needs with an artificial supplement.

Large doses of otherwise good nutrients can cause health problems. Excessive vitamin D can cause symptoms ranging from nausea to kidney failure. Too much vitamin A can lead to headaches, hair loss, and liver damage. Avoid taking supplements that contain more than the U.S. recommended daily allowance (USRDA) of any nutrient.

Another reason whole foods are superior to supplements is the availability of the nutrients to your body. It's not enough for a pill to contain 100 percent of your daily vitamin and mineral needs if those nutrients are provided in a form your body can't easily use. The availability of nutrients is sometimes strongly affected by the presence of other nutrients. A multivitamin and mineral pill contains ingredients that get in each other's way. For instance, high doses of iron will interfere with your body's ability to absorb zinc and copper.

That's not to say you shouldn't take a daily supplement, but a pill is not a fix for poor eating habits. Think of vitamin and mineral pills as a way to increase your chances of getting all the nutrients you need. Your prenatal supplement is a good source of nutrients that might help to fill in the blanks on your body's nutritional checklist. Avoid taking any additional supplements without the approval of your health care provider.

Breastmilk and Your Diet

When you eat a rich, varied diet, your baby enjoys a variety of milk flavors. Today, it's a creamy garlic sauce courtesy of last night's Italian dinner. Tomorrow, who knows? Your baby will get her first exposure to the foods you like through the flavor of your milk.

Foods to Avoid

Most women can eat anything they want while breastfeeding without any problems. However, there are some foods that have a bad reputation among nursing mothers. These foods can pass into your breastmilk and change its flavor or cause allergic reactions in your baby. Symptoms vary but usually involve fussiness, an unwillingness to nurse, rash, diarrhea, or vomiting. Often, a baby who suddenly refuses to nurse is responding to the flavor of your milk. If your baby displays any of these symptoms, examine your diet and check it against this list of the usual suspects.

- Caffeine
- Chocolate
- Citrus fruits
- Dairy products
- Foods that cause gas
- Nuts (especially peanuts)
- Spicy foods

Eliminating these foods from your diet might help. However, the change in your baby will not be immediate. To find the offending food, try cutting out one of the possible culprits from your diet for a week or two. If your baby's symptoms persist, try eliminating the next food.

A recent Canadian study found that women who eat peanuts have detectable amounts of peanut proteins in their breastmilk. These proteins can sensitize a baby to peanuts, leading to a potentially fatal allergic reaction when the child is older and eats peanut products.

Once you identify a problem food, keep it off your menu for a few months. Older babies can more easily tolerate a variety of flavors. Another solution is to avoid large amounts of any one food at a time. Some women find they are able to eat small amounts of their problem foods if they don't do it very often. No two women are the same, so you'll have to experiment a little.

Healthy Snacks

It's not always easy to prepare regular meals with a new baby in the house. Luckily, good nutrition is just as easy to achieve by "grazing" as it is by eating three square meals every day. Keeping healthy snacks on hand is a great way to get your RDAs, keep off unwanted weight, and set a good lifelong example for your child. Instead of chips or cookies, try some of the following quick and healthy alternatives or add your own from the Food Pyramid.

- Apples
- Bananas
- Breads
- Cantaloupe
- Carrot sticks
- Celery
- Cereal
- Crackers
- Eggs
- Grapes
- Oranges
- Plums
- Popcorn (plain)
- Salads
- Soups
- Strawberries
- Tomatoes (may cause gas)
- Yogurt

Special Concerns

Whether you're a vegetarian or have medical restrictions, you'll want to take extra care. Special attention is important not only for your baby's nutrition, but also to preserve your own health. If you need additional information, consult your doctor or a nutritionist.

Vegetarian Diet

If you're a vegetarian, you already pay special attention to your diet. Lacto-ovo vegetarians, who eat eggs and dairy products, can generally meet all their nutritional needs from food sources. However, vegans, those vegetarians who don't eat any animal products at all, are at risk for nutritional deficiencies in several important areas. Protein, vitamin D, riboflavin, calcium, iron, and zinc are harder to find in plant form than in animal products, but it can be done.

VITAMINS	
B_{12}	fortified soy beverages and cereals
D	fortified soy beverages and sunshine
Riboflavin (B_2)	fortified whole grains, avocados, and nuts
MINERALS	
Calcium	soy beverages, calcium-enriched orange juice, broccoli, nuts, seeds, bok choy, greens, grains, peas and beans, kale, and some tofus
Iron	green leafy vegetables, iron-fortified cereals and breads, peas, beans, tofu, dried fruits, and whole grains
Zinc	tofu, nuts, peas, beans, wheat germ, bran, whole grain breads
PROTEINS	SOY, NUTS, SEEDS, PEAS, BEANS, GRAINS, AND VEGETABLES

Vitamin B_{12} does not naturally occur in plant sources, and vegans, lactating or not, need to supplement this important nutrient. The continued use of a prenatal vitamin and mineral supplement while nursing is an especially good idea for vegetarian mothers.

There is also some question about the availability of important, brain-nourishing fats like DHA in strict vegan diets. Noted pediatric experts Martha and William Sears believe so strongly in the importance of DHA in a breastfeeding mom's diet that they recommend vegans temporarily add fish to their daily menu. Consider the following suggestions of good dietary sources for the nutrients most often lacking in vegetarian diets.

Teen Moms

Mothers below the age of nineteen are still growing and have more nutritional needs than older moms. The U.S. Department of Agriculture (USDA) recommends additional calcium, phosphorus, and magnesium for teen moms. Phosphorus works with calcium to form teeth and bones. Magnesium is necessary in the production of healthy bones, teeth, and nerves. Magnesium also helps prevent heart attacks and stroke. Teen mothers should make special efforts to incorporate the following into their diet:

- Calcium: Milk, cheese, whole grains, egg yolk, peas, beans, nuts, green leafy vegetables
- Phosphorus: Milk, cheese, meat, egg yolk, whole grains, peas, beans, nuts
- Magnesium: dark green leafy vegetables, bananas, dried apricots, avocados, cashews, almonds, soy products, whole grains, chocolate

In addition to focusing on the previous elements, very young mothers should be diligent about taking their prenatal vitamins and having regular OB visits.

Weight-Loss Plans

Breastfeeding is a wonderful, natural weight-loss plan. Studies consistently show that women who nurse their babies return to their prepregnancy weight faster than moms who formula feed. All the fat cells your body stockpiled during pregnancy, and even some from before, will be used to make milk for your baby.

When you breastfeed, your body needs about 500 extra calories every day. That means you can eat a little bit more than usual and still lose weight. If you only consume an extra 300 calories every day, your body will use your fat stores to make up the difference.

Changes in your diet can pose a risk to your health if you have certain preexisting medical conditions. If you are on a restricted diet of any kind, talk with your health care provider before making any changes. Even a vitamin and mineral pill can cause problems for some people.

Your weight loss while breastfeeding will be slow but steady. That's the way nature intended it. Crash dieting puts you at risk for nutritional deficiencies and might eventually affect the quality of your milk. Besides, crash diets don't work. Studies show that rapid weight loss at any time of life is usually followed by rapid weight gain. The best way to keep weight off is to lose it gradually through a combination of diet and exercise.

Choosing healthy foods and drinking lots of water during lactation will get you into the right habits. Keep your weight loss down to one pound per week or less. Even half a pound per week will melt away those pregnancy pounds within a year.

CHAPTER 15

Exercise for You and Your Baby

How can exercise affect breast-feeding? Anything that helps a nursing mother stay confident and ward off depression also helps her have a positive breastfeeding experience. Your mind and body have far-reaching effects on each other, and that connection can make all the difference in the quality of your life. It's vital to realize that exercise is not only compatible with lactation, it's beneficial as well.

The Benefits of Exercise

This might not feel like the best time to start or resume a program of exercise, but exercise can help you in every part of your life, including breastfeeding. As little as twenty to thirty minutes of aerobic exercise three or four times per week can help you feel better, look better, and live longer. Toning exercises like sit-ups and leg lifts can help your body regain its prepregnancy shape more quickly. Any amount of exercise will burn up calories and help you lose some of that leftover pregnancy weight.

Exercise

- Increases your energy level
- Steps up your metabolism so you burn more calories even at rest
- Tones your muscles
- Gives you a sense of accomplishment that boosts your confidence
- Improves your circulation
- Fights off depression and boredom
- Helps you to lose weight
- Makes you feel sexier

As important as exercise is, don't overdo it! Weight loss should be very gradual in breastfeeding women. One pound per week is the maximum. If you're losing more than that, you're putting yourself and your baby at risk for nutritional deficiencies. Exercise for health, not just weight loss.

Remember to always stretch before and after a workout. Stretching lengthens your muscles, increases your flexibility, and greatly reduces your chance of injury. You'll also find stretching helpful in relieving muscle cramps and other muscle-related pains.

When to Begin

Always get your doctor's approval before beginning an exercise program. There are conditions, like Caesarean section delivery and abdominal diastasis, that might keep you more sedentary than you would like.

Adequate recovery time and sometimes specialized exercise routines are absolute necessities to avoid dangerous complications.

Doctors generally advise women without special conditions to wait at least six weeks after delivery before beginning or resuming an aerobic exercise program. Your body needs the time both to recover from childbearing and to establish a good milk supply. You and your baby also need those first weeks to work out a nursing routine.

QUESTIONS?

What is abdominal diastasis?
Labor may cause a separation of the vertical muscles in your abdomen, called diastasis, and even mild exertion can make it worse.

However, that doesn't mean you're on bed rest. Shaping and toning exercises are generally all right. Sit-ups and leg lifts can help your body recover. You can also go about any normal activity that doesn't cause you pain or undue stress. Walking is a great all-around exercise anytime. Just take it slow and work your way up to the level of activity you want.

Finding the Time

With all the new responsibilities of parenthood, clearing your schedule at a certain time every day for exercise isn't always practical. It's easy to get so busy that you forget to take care of yourself. Everyone else's needs seem to come first. Your baby needs to be fed, changed, and held. Your toddler needs attention, stimulation, and socialization. The dog needs to be walked. In those busy first months, you've got to become an exercise opportunist.

Make exercise part of your ordinary activities. Three ten-minute chunks of time are as effective as thirty minutes in a row. Shorter stretches are easier to get through and easier to schedule. Even little activities that seem like they wouldn't make much of a difference add up quickly over the course of a few months.

- Sit up five or ten times in the morning when you first get up from bed. Add an extra sit-up every few days.

- Use the stairs instead of the escalator.
- Park at the far end of the parking lot.
- Choose to stand instead of sit.
- Flex your muscles and hold them tight while you sit in traffic.
- Run in place.
- Tighten Kegel muscles just about anywhere.
- Tackle the housework. Laundry, dishes, taking out the garbage, washing windows, and vacuuming the floor are productive workouts.
- Do the yard work. Let your husband watch the baby while you weed, mow, or shovel.

After you and your baby have negotiated a sleep schedule, you can start to enjoy more traditional workouts a few times per week. It's hard for new parents to imagine having the time for a formal workout, but remember that exercise only seems like it takes time. It really saves time.

Exercise sharpens both your mind and body, helping you cut through your tasks more quickly with less effort. The little bit of time you spend on exercise will pay you back many times over with increased efficiency.

Your Changing Body

During pregnancy, your body went through some major changes. Lactation adds new and different demands. Your body isn't the same as it was before pregnancy, and you've got to keep that in mind as you exercise.

The American College of Obstetricians and Gynecologists has issued guidelines for exercise during the weeks after childbirth.

1. Exercise regularly, at least three times per week. If you're playing a sport, don't compete.
2. Don't exercise too hard in hot, humid weather.
3. Keep your movements smooth. Don't bounce or jerk. Exercise on a wooden floor or a tightly carpeted surface.
4. Your joints are looser than normal, so avoid flexing or extending them very far. Loose joints can lead to dislocation or damage, so avoid jumping, jarring, or rapid changes in direction.

5. Always warm up for five minutes before any vigorous workout. Slow walking is a good warm-up.

6. At the end of a workout, slow down gradually and stretch. However, because your joints are looser than normal, don't stretch any joint to its maximum position.

7. Women should monitor their heart rates and stay within the range advised by their doctors.

8. Rise slowly. There's an increased risk of fainting due to sudden changes in your blood pressure. Work your legs gently for a few minutes after you get back on your feet.

9. Drink plenty of water to avoid dehydration. Drink whenever you're thirsty, even if it means interrupting the workout.

10. If you haven't been very active in the past, you should start slowly and increase your workout over time.

11. At the first sign of unusual symptoms, you should stop exercising and contact your doctor.

Lactating moms need to take some other precautions as well. Nurse your baby or express your milk before working out and wear a good, supportive sports bra. Full breasts can be painful if they are jostled around too much.

After a workout, immediately remove your bra. Wash your breasts with plain water and let them air dry. A sweaty breast might be unappealingly salty to your baby, and clean, dry breasts are much less likely to become infected from clogged milk ducts.

Exercise and Breastmilk

Over the last few years, many of us have heard reports that exercise sours breastmilk and leads to fussy babies that reject the breast. This is simply not true. All the speculation is based on a single study that compared breastmilk samples taken before and after exhaustive exercise sessions.

In that study, it was observed that babies seemed less eager to take breastmilk immediately after their moms had worked out to near exhaustion. Researchers blamed lactic acid, a normal by-product of exercise, for the effect. That's as much information as most of the public received. Less known is that the effect lasted for only about one hour. So, if your exercise routine involves pushing on to the point of exhaustion, you might want to wait an hour before feeding your child. Otherwise, you really don't need to worry about any negative effects to your milk.

Exercises to Do with Your Baby

Involving your baby or toddler in your exercise routine makes working out fun and it's a great way to get closer to your child.

- Put your baby in a sling or a stroller and go for a long family walk. You can walk through the park, around the mall, or just around your neighborhood.
- Buy a jogging stroller with big bicycle tires and take your child on a run.
- Buy a bike trailer and take him for a ride.
- Pull your toddler behind you in a wagon.
- Do sit-ups in front of your baby in a bouncy swing, and say "peek-a-boo" every time you come forward. She'll love it!
- Lie on the floor next to your baby and do leg lifts. It's a great way to exercise while still maintaining face-to-face contact.
- Dance with your child in your arms—slow or fast or anywhere in between.
- Use your baby as a weight. When she is old enough to support her head, lift her up while you're lying on the floor. Bring her to your nose with a smile and some words of love, then put her back out at arm's length and do it again.

Toddlers can be a workout all by themselves. Just try to keep up with yours for a while! If you really want a workout, take your toddler to the home of a friend who doesn't have children. People without kids always have lots of breakable things within a toddler's easy reach. By the time you've followed two steps behind your curious youngster for an hour, you'll feel like you've run a marathon.

CHAPTER 16

Stress, Postpartum Depression, and Breastfeeding

Yes, your life has changed! Happy events like moving or starting a new job can cause stress, and having a new baby is a major life adjustment. Learning to parent a newborn might be both the happiest time in your life as well as the most stressful. Now is the time to have friends and family present to share in this joyous time, and to support you in your new role.

"Discontented Cows Don't Give Milk"

Suzanne recently spoke to the wife of a dairy farmer. She was told that dairy cows are made to feel as comfortable as possible in order to produce an abundant milk supply. They eat, sleep, and give milk, and that's all that's expected of them. Don't all new mothers wish life were that simple! When women come to lactation consultants with problems relating to plugged ducts, mastitis, and milk supply, in essence, that is the advice they are given. Eat, sleep, and give milk.

Stress and Your Milk Supply

Stress can affect your milk supply to some degree, but every woman is different. Some women who live in war-torn countries or who suffer from severe malnutrition can still supply enough milk to keep their babies well nourished. Other mothers don't fare as well. While the baby's demand will regulate your milk production, a stressed mother and a fussy baby are likely to threaten the success of the breastfeeding relationship.

FACTS

Increased smoking and nicotine levels can impact your milk supply. Smokers who are stressed tend to smoke more and inhale more deeply. If you are smoking more than a pack a day, you might experience a reduction in both your milk supply and your letdown.

Stress and fatigue cause an increase in adrenaline levels in the body, and adrenaline is a major inhibitor in the production of oxytocin. Oxytocin commands the letdown reflex. When you're stressed, you might have a repressed letdown, which means that your baby must work harder to get milk from your breast. The harder he has to work, the more frustrated he becomes. This sets the stage for a difficult breastfeeding experience, and without intervention, it might end the beginning of a beautiful relationship.

An Ounce of Prevention

There are several ways to encourage relaxation and inner calm. One possible solution is creative visualization, which has been shown to

improve milk supply. Camomile tea has been used for centuries as a mild sedative and is safe for nursing women. Lavender oil on your pillowcase or massaged into your temples will help you relax and let your milk down. Breast massage before and during a feeding session is also beneficial.

Remember to nurse often and to focus on your baby. During the first few weeks, you're negotiating a nursing routine with your newborn. Frequent nursing will guarantee the maintenance of your milk supply. You might find breastfeeding stressful, but after your routine is established, it will be some of the best time you spend with your baby.

Sleep Deprivation

Being the parent of a newborn is like experiencing an altered state of consciousness. Many factors seem to work against your ability to get a good night's sleep. Midnight feedings, regulating your sleep cycle to match your baby's, and recovering from labor anesthesia all take their toll. Those stresses can create a surreal feeling of walking in a haze those first few days after the birth of your infant.

Many experts, friends, and family will tell new mothers to sleep when their baby sleeps. This piece of sage advice is priceless. Housework can wait, but your mental health cannot. Sleep as often as you can, or call a friend to baby-sit so you can rest soundly. Preserving your sleep time requires putting your baby to bed. Sometimes we are so caught up with gazing at their angelic faces in slumber that we hold them throughout their naps, but you'll have lots of opportunities to bond. For now, let sleeping babies lie. Other strategies include taking turns with your spouse or assigning shifts at night.

The Baby Blues

In the fourth century, Hippocrates, the Father of Physicians, discovered a condition he called "puerperal fever." It was believed that "suppressed lochial discharge" (the discharge following birth) inflamed the brain and caused delirium and manic attacks. An eleventh-century gynecologist,

Trotula of Salerno, thought that "if the womb is moist, the brain is filled with water, and the moisture running over the eyes compels women to involuntarily shed tears." Even in the eighteenth century, a book by a physician named Marce was entitled, "Treatice on Insanity in Pregnant and Lactating Women." Although these men were onto something, their definitions were scientifically suspect and politically incorrect by today's standards. In the spirit of the day, however, this was an important acknowledgment that the baby blues is a very real condition.

Almost 50 to 90 percent of women experience some form of the baby blues. These tearful, weepy days usually begin about three to five days following birth, as hormones rapidly change in response to the loss of the placenta. Sleep deprivation, lack of confidence in parenting a newborn, isolation from the outside world, and the 24/7 demands of a new baby serve only to compound these feelings.

QUESTIONS?

How can hypothyroidism affect your milk supply?
Hypothyroidism occurs when the thyroid gland fails to produce a sufficient amount of its hormone. That hormone regulates your metabolism and can cause a reduction in your milk supply. Symptoms can include nervousness, sweating, increased heart palpitations, upset stomach, diarrhea, and weight loss. A physical exam by your doctor will diagnose or rule out this condition in relationship to postpartum depression.

The blues are characterized by feelings of inadequacy, exhaustion, confusion, euphoria, insomnia, and mood swings. Because the vast majority of women experience some of these symptoms, this condition is considered normal. The baby blues are also considered transient. These feelings usually disappear within the first two weeks following birth, and sometimes they go away within hours of when they began.

Most women tend to muddle through, have a good cry to release some tension, or seek support from a strong husband or good friend. However, if your mood doesn't improve by your baby's two-week checkup, or if your feelings seem overwhelming, tell your health care

provider. He or she might provide some additional testing or refer you to a counselor. The baby blues can lead to postpartum depression (PPD), a much more serious condition.

Stress-Stopping Toolbox

Things that seem so obvious are truly innovative for new, breastfeeding mothers engrossed in taking care of their babies. Ways to relax and take care of yourself may be the farthest thing from your mind, but remember that your physical and mental health is critical to successful breastfeeding and parenting. With that in mind, remember to do at least a few of the following every day:

Breathe. Lie on your bed and take deep abdominal cleansing breaths. Focus on your breathing. Try yoga.

Eat right and eat light. High-protein foods like nuts, seeds, and beans will increase your energy level. So will iron-rich foods like eggs, red meat, fish, poultry, whole grain cereals and breads, dried fruits, and legumes. Drink a glass of orange juice with these. Vitamin C helps your body absorb iron more efficiently. Iron will help you combat fatigue and anemia. Prepare handy "grab-it" baggies of baby carrots, pretzels, or grapes. They'll be ready when you are for a quick snack break.

Exercise. Your body releases endorphins after several minutes of exercise. Endorphins are your body's natural painkillers. They also make you feel good about yourself and are considered a natural high. Put your newborn in a stroller and walk around the block.

Laugh! Rent a funny movie, read a humor book, or talk to a friend who makes you giggle. Laughter is indeed the best medicine!

Massage. A good massage reduces the stress hormone known as cortisol. It also boosts your immune system, alleviates stress, helps you relax, and induces sleep. And it feels so good! Long, slow strokes that follow the growth of hair follicles (downward motions) relax the body, while strokes that go against hair growth (upward motions) stimulate your body. Remember to avoid direct pressure on the spine when giving massage.

Prioritize. Is it more important to take care of yourself or your laundry? This is a very busy time for you. Think about what really matters most. Now that you are a family, work may have to wait. Don't let someone else's crisis be your own. Slow down and reprioritize your goals.

ESSENTIALS

Find a sitter so you can go to a movie, take a walk, read a book, or shop. Do those things you enjoyed before your baby arrived. You need time to re-energize yourself, too!

Sleep. There is no better way to re-energize than to take catnaps whenever possible. Sleep when your baby sleeps. Or better yet, lie down together and breastfeed. Develop bedtime rituals for yourself and your baby. Bath, book, bed. As a new parent, you probably won't have any trouble falling asleep, but if you do, try eating healthy bedtime snacks that induce sleep, like a slice of turkey on a bagel with a glass of warm milk.

Take vitamins. Your prenatal vitamins contain minerals like magnesium, folic acid, and zinc. Those, coupled with B and C vitamins, will help maintain your body's energy. Vitamins alone can't accomplish what a healthy, balanced diet can, so use these in conjunction with nutritious foods.

Talk. Your frustrations are real. Call a friend, a parent, or a crisis line, if needed. Join a moms' group. Develop new support systems with people who have previous experience in parenting. Surround yourself with positive people.

Try black walnuts. Black walnut teas, supplements, and meats boost serotonin levels and combat depression.

Use aromatherapy. Add a few drops of jasmine, clary sage, lavender, or rose oil to your bath or bed pillow. These scents have been shown to reduce stress and induce relaxation.

Walk. Fresh air can work wonders for a distressed spirit.

Taking care of yourself sometimes means simply going easy on yourself. Be mindful of your expectations, especially the universal one:

Somehow you will be the perfect parent. As you know, no one is perfect and no one can do it all, at least not for long. Don't set yourself up to fail, and don't sweat the small stuff. Realistic expectations can decrease your risk for PPD and relieve your anxiety.

Postpartum Depression

When the baby blues extends beyond what is considered the normal two-week period, it may turn into a more serious condition called postpartum depression, or PPD.

- PPD affects 10 to 30 percent of all new mothers. The number of teen and single parents with this condition is even higher.
- If left untreated, 25 percent of women will still suffer from the symptoms up to one year later.
- The onset of PPD usually occurs within the first six weeks after birth.

PPD is characterized by feelings of listlessness, frequent crying, insomnia, anger, sadness, headaches, anxiety attacks, and a sense of hopelessness. Take the quiz below to see how you score on the scale.

Postpartum Depression Quiz

Since the birth of your baby, have you experienced . . .

- ❑ Loss of interest in usually pleasurable activities?
- ❑ Difficulty concentrating or making decisions?
- ❑ Changes in appetite and/or sleep?
- ❑ Excessive anxiety over your baby's health?
- ❑ Feelings of worthlessness or guilt, especially feelings of failure as a mother?
- ❑ Fatigue?
- ❑ Excessive, repetitive, or nervous nonproductive activity like pacing, fidgeting, or an inability to sit still?
- ❑ A lack of desire to care for yourself, your infant, or your family?
- ❑ Recurrent thoughts of death or suicide?

If you answered yes to four or more of these questions, you could be diagnosed with PPD. Contact your health care provider immediately and take this test with you. You don't have to feel alone. There is help available right now!

What Causes PPD and How Is It Treated?

No one is certain what causes PPD, but most experts agree that many factors play a role.

During pregnancy, hormones like estrogen, progesterone, prolactin, and cortisol, as well as ovarian steroids, interact to maintain a healthy pregnancy. After the delivery of the placenta, these hormone levels rapidly decline. Some alter central nervous system responses like memory, movement, language, emotions, thought processes, and involuntary body processes. The central nervous system is also important in the regulation of attention, sleep, and arousal.

There is also a clear connection between a family history of depression and PPD. If you have previously been diagnosed with depression, tell your doctor. The risk of having PPD with a second baby is one hundred times greater if you've had it before.

Women with poor or abusive relationships, who lack support, and suffer child care stress have an increased risk of PPD. Women with prior histories of depression, panic disorder, obsessive-compulsive disorder, premenstrual syndrome, or previous PPD episodes are at the greatest risk. Notify your health care provider immediately.

PPD is generally treated in three phases. Medications like Zoloft, Prozac, Paxil, or tricyclic antidepressants, safe for breastfeeding mothers, are widely used to treat symptoms in the first six to twelve weeks following diagnosis. Tricyclic antidepressants are commonly used with lactating women because there are fewer side effects in the infants of treated mothers. Prozac can cause some weight loss and takes longer for your body to shed, so this is a medication of last resort, but it's still possible to nurse while using this drug.

SSENTIALS

Multiple births present increased challenges to your mental health. With the loss of their one supersized placenta or two smaller ones, mothers of multiples experience a more massive shift in hormones than other mothers. This puts them at a greater risk for PPD.

Although PPD is a serious condition, it is treatable. The condition itself is outside your control, but you do have control to take steps toward recovery. You're not alone and shouldn't have to suffer by yourself. Locate mental health professionals in your community who specialize in postpartum disorders. Call your health care provider or contact your local United Way, WIC office, Visiting Nurse Services, or maternal/child health organization for referrals to individuals who can assist you. Remember, seeking help when you need it is a sign of strength, not a weakness.

PPD and Breastfeeding

When diagnosed with PPD, many women are told to wean their babies in order to be treated with antidepressants, but this is not always the best course of action. Weaning can compound feelings of depression by further reducing your body's production of prolactin. In fact, in many women, symptoms of PPD don't appear until weaning begins.

Prolactin is the hormone responsible for initiating milk production. It's also nature's built-in tranquilizer for nursing mothers. Prolactin levels in your body increase when your baby suckles. Perhaps not coincidentally, PPD is often diagnosed at six weeks postpartum, the time when many women must return to work and have prepared to end their exclusive breastfeeding relationship.

Some depressed mothers often fail to respond appropriately to their infant's cues to feed, or might allow others to offer formula because they are simply unmotivated to breastfeed. Both of these situations can have devastating effects on both your infant and your milk supply. Babies of depressed mothers sometimes develop depression, too. Seek assistance from your health care provider if you suspect your baby might be affected by your depression.

FACTS

Studies indicate that women who have active support present during their labor and delivery have fewer reported episodes of PPD. Although some women might have more support at home than you have, there are steps you can take to enjoy a less stressful labor and delivery. Doulas, spouses, family, and friends are available to make your birthing experience more positive. Contact DONA for more information.

If you've been diagnosed with PPD, you can continue to breastfeed. As long as your medications are safe, you can nurse your baby. Your doctor will prescribe the minimum effective dose and will monitor your infant throughout the process.

Resources for PPD

Be sure to tell your health care provider if your baby blues extend beyond the first two weeks after your baby's birth. Their goal is to develop a health history with you, so they need to know what sources of support are available and what services you've tried.

The following organizations are in place to help you work through feelings and other symptoms associated with PPD.

Center for Pre and Postpartum Disorders	609-497-1144
Depression after Delivery	800-944-4PPD
Mother Risk Toronto	416-813-6780
Postpartum Education for Parents Warmline	805-564-3888
Postpartum Stress Center	610-525-7527
Postpartum Support International	805-967-7636
Pregnancy and Postpartum Treatment	312-996-2972

Support from Family and Friends

In many cultures, extended family and women kin attend the birth of the baby, then keep watch over mother and infant for up to thirty days following delivery, and sometimes longer. This kith-and-kin network offers parents a chance to get to know their babies without the stress of having to do all the chores of life like meal preparation and house cleaning.

The American Way

The extended family socialization of other cultures has worked for centuries for many reasons. In addition to the "many hands make light work" element, friends and family provide much-needed emotional support for new parents. These communities have fewer reported cases of PPD because they offer support throughout the time when family adjustment is most critical.

In our society, we operate a little differently. While mothers and mothers-in-law often come to stay for a week or so, women feel more inclined to entertain them as guests, rather than to accept their assistance. If this is the case for you, it is important to limit the number of visitors who come to call during the first few weeks after your baby arrives. If you have a hard time saying no, ask your husband to screen your phone calls or simply say, "I'd like to have you over once things settle down a bit. I appreciate your patience and look forward to seeing you."

Use Your Resources

If you can truly use the support your friends offer, then by all means, accept it! There are several different types of support and we need them all: emotional, informational, tangible, and social.

Knowledge is power—Informational support is the easiest to access. When we have questions, we read a book, search the Web, call an expert, or ask a friend. However, other types of support can be more difficult to obtain.

Open up!—Sharing intimate moments with people who care about you and understand you facilitates emotional support. Your husband, best friend, and family are there for you, to listen and provide advice and encouragement. This kind of support is extremely valuable if you suffer from symptoms of PPD or stress. Your loved ones genuinely want to help and will be there when you call.

Gift horses—Tangible support comes by way of baby-sitting offers, diapers and supplies, cash assistance, or rides to the grocery store. There might be times when this help is desperately needed. Keep these offers open-ended for when they come in handy.

Network—Social support includes groups of people who can provide assistance in a general way, like your health care provider, La Leche League, and your colleagues and other acquaintances. The help they offer can take the form of participation in groups and programs, or individual services based on your particular needs.

Asking for support takes a certain amount of bravery, but it will come more easily each time your call is answered. Concentrate on one helper with one task for one time. The goal is to seek assistance over the first few weeks of your baby's life.

QUESTIONS?

What can a dad do if his wife suffers from PPD?
Your patience and encouragement are loving ways to communicate your support for her. Listen to her feelings and try to understand her. Don't blame her for something outside of her control. Take care of your baby as best you can, and don't ignore your own feelings—you are important, too!

Remember, too, that relationships are based on give-and-take. After your life has settled down and you are in a comfortable routine, you can pay back these favors one at a time. Most people find great satisfaction in helping others. Welcome the chance to return favors when the time comes.

CHAPTER 17

Sex and the Breastfeeding Couple

American culture loves to emphasize the sexuality of the breasts. Conversely, some people, even health care professionals, want to desexualize the breast entirely. They point out that breasts are clearly designed to feed babies and that's serious business. Your breasts are wonderful sources of nourishment and emotional comfort for your baby, but they're sexual, too. Your challenge is to find the balance that works for you and your partner.

The Great Sexuality Debate

People who want to desexualize breasts are usually reacting to the way sexuality can interfere with breastfeeding. For instance, some husbands find it difficult at first to share their partner's breasts with a baby. They might be unwilling to accommodate any other use for their private playground. It seems like everything from public nursing to our most private thoughts and feelings about breastfeeding can get all tangled up in our attitudes about sex.

Let's state right here that, yes, breasts are sexual—but your whole body is sexual. When it comes to making a body part sexual, it's in the way that you use it. In many cultures, breasts are just one more piece of a woman's anatomy, like an arm or a leg. There are cultures (and individuals) that find a well-turned ankle, the eyes, or even a quick mind far more exciting than an exposed breast.

QUESTIONS?

Do some women feel aroused while breastfeeding?
It's normal for some women to become sexually aroused while breastfeeding. Oxytocin, the hormone released by your body when baby suckles, is also released during sex. Some women even reach orgasm. Breastfeeding is a pleasurable experience. It's one of nature's rewards.

Speaking of minds, the brain is your most important sexual organ. Sex is a combination of friction and fantasy. For some men, part of the thrill of breasts is the context in which they have access to them. If your husband is one of these guys, he might only be used to seeing your breasts during sexual encounters.

So, now are your breasts only for the baby? No, not if you're comfortable with breast play as a part of your sexual relationship with your mate. Your breasts can be less sensitive, overly sensitive, or unchanged in the weeks following birth. All of these conditions are normal. If you enjoy the contact, there's no reason you can't resume breast play.

Changing Relationships

Before your baby was born, the relationship you enjoyed with your partner took center stage in your life. You were lovers, friends, and playmates. Now, you're Mom and Dad. For some people, it's difficult to reconcile these new roles with the old ones. Some men believe that their wife's new status as mother makes her untouchable.

Guys like that need a little reminder that their mates are still sexual beings. Are mothers sexy? You bet they are! Mothers are women, not girls. They have given birth. They're fertile and sensuous. If you're ready for sex but your husband doesn't seem interested, make the first move. Most men love that. It might be just the thing he needs to jog his memory about how you became parents in the first place.

ESSENTIALS

Most women experience a lack of interest in sex following the birth of their baby. Hormonal changes serve to focus a new mother's attention where nature wants it, on the baby. It's a temporary condition, but combined with sleep deprivation, it can leave little room for romance.

Nursing your baby is a wonderfully satisfying, intimate experience. You might even come to feel that your body belongs first to your baby, and second to your husband. Your hormone levels while lactating can contribute to those feelings. Estrogen levels are low and that affects your desire for sex as well as the amount of natural lubrication produced by your vagina. It's as if nature was saying, "You've got a baby. You don't need sex until it's time for another one."

Although your sexual needs might have temporarily changed, your partner's needs are nearly the same as they've always been. He might be a little less amorous than usual because of the exhaustion that's common to all new parents, but he still looks forward to spending time alone with you. That doesn't mean you have to supply him with sex on demand, just try to stay connected emotionally. One way is to keep your mate involved in your most important activity, the care of your child.

You might not feel that your partner knows what he's doing when he tries to help out, but resist the urge to correct your husband when he changes a diaper or attempts to comfort your crying child. It's vital that your mate bonds with your baby, too. You're not just nurturing a child, you're nurturing a family.

The two of you are in this thing together, and you need each other now more than you ever have before. Your lives have changed and they won't be getting back to "normal." It's up to you and your partner to find a new "normal" for your relationship. Give her the support she needs to be a good mother. If you find yourself doing more around the house, don't think in terms of "I'm helping her out." Your life together is a partnership. Court her to remind her that she's the love of your life. A loving relationship with your wife is one of the best gifts you can give your baby. Stay intimate in a hundred little ways and don't pressure her for sex. You'll both feel bad about it later.

Intimacy

Intimacy doesn't mean sex. Rather, true intimacy is a matter of the mind. It's simply knowing and caring about your partner's thoughts, needs, and feelings, but mostly it's about trust. Trust that you'll be there when you're needed, trust that you'll love your partner no matter what, and trust that you can be yourself with each other. The two of you are pulling together as a team.

Where there's true intimacy between a couple, sex follows naturally. Until you're both ready for physical intimacy, you can stay connected with your partner in many simple, nonsexual ways.

- Leave love notes around the house for your mate.
- Take a walk together.
- Surprise your partner with a gift. It doesn't have to be anything big, just a little way of saying, "I'm thinking of you."
- Say "I love you" and mean it.

- Go on a date. Take a deep breath and hire that baby-sitter. Go to your favorite restaurant or have a picnic. It's all right to talk about the baby. It might be hard to think about anything else at first. Your child is the focus of your life right now, but don't let that one topic dominate the conversation.
- Laugh together.
- Help out around the house.
- Take an interest in the activities your mate enjoys.
- Give a massage. A breastfeeding mom is especially prone to sore back and shoulders. You can even rub her feet while she nurses the baby.
- Look your best. Often, you just need to be comfortable around your home and sweatpants and a T-shirt are fine. On occasion, though, treat your spouse to the glamorous version of you that's usually reserved for special events. Making yourself attractive for your partner shows them how important they are to you.
- Write a love song or rewrite the words to an existing song. Your song can be dripping with romance or it can be funny. As an alternative, make a tape or CD of the songs that are special to the two of you.
- Give up some minor habit you know annoys your mate. Tapping your fingers or putting your elbows on the table might seem like minor issues, but changing your behavior out of love is a major gesture.

Through it all, communicate. Talk about everything. It's especially important to discuss your feelings before a problem develops. Use the phrase "I feel . . ." instead of assuming that your feelings are an accurate measure of the situation.

If you can communicate openly and respectfully with each other, you'll find that you share many of the same thoughts and fears. Together, you can reach much more mutually satisfying solutions than you ever could apart. Keeping the lines of communication open will even help with those situations where all you can do is endure. Labor, exhaustion, colic, and a new parent's fears are all easier to take when you have a hand to hold and a shoulder to cry on.

Sex

Most American doctors advise new parents to wait at least six weeks after birth before having sex. In other countries, a three-week wait is standard. In any case, your body needs some time to heal. The separation in your uterine lining caused by the expulsion of the placenta must close and tears or episiotomy incisions have to heal and become flexible again. Six weeks might not be enough time for all of that to happen.

FACTS

Numbers and norms vary among women, but research has clearly shown that breastfeeding speeds recovery from pregnancy and childbirth. A faster recovery would seem to naturally favor a more immediate return to sexual readiness.

Breastfeeding might also have an influence on how quickly women resume sex, but it's difficult to tell based on current research. One study reported that breastfeeding couples tend to wait a little longer than other couples. Another study reported that breastfeeding moms resumed sexual relations not only sooner than other moms, but enjoyed it more and experienced less pain. In agreement, yet another study suggests that women who breastfeed return to arousability sooner than women who don't breastfeed.

The Big Day

Eventually, you'll feel ready for intercourse. That first time after childbirth is a lot like your other first time. The experience can be anywhere from mildly uncomfortable to downright painful. When you're ready to give it a try, you'll need to take a few special precautions.

Relax. In her popular book, *The Girlfriends' Guide to Surviving the First Year of Motherhood*, Vicki McCarty Lovine recommends that you "inebriate and lubricate." That advice might work for some women, but breastfeeding mothers need to be careful about using a glass of wine or any other alcoholic beverage to help them relax. Whenever you plan to have a drink, nurse your baby first, and allow at least one hour to pass for every drink you consume before breastfeeding your baby again. If you feed your baby and then have two glasses of wine, you should wait at least two hours from the last drink. Most new moms are exhausted and alcohol can send them right to sleep.

Pay attention to lubrication. Postpartum estrogen levels reduce your vagina's natural lubrication, so have a tube of the artificial stuff on hand. K-Y jelly and Astroglide are good choices. Spermicidal jellies are another. Normal amounts of lubrication usually return after your first menstrual cycle.

Use birth control. You might need to try a different method than usual while breastfeeding. Consult the sections on fertility and birth control below for advice.

Let her lead. Women generally prefer to be on top or lie side-by-side with their husband (the spoon position) during intercourse. These positions let you control the amount of pressure put on delicate perineal tissue.

Communicate. Moms, let your husband know what you enjoy and what's just too uncomfortable right now. Don't suffer through the event. Your partner wants you to enjoy yourself. That might be a tall order the first few times, but at a minimum, you shouldn't have to be in pain. If you decide to grin and bear it, you're just going to be even more nervous about sex in the future. That can lead to a loss of intimacy with your partner if you become afraid that loving attention will lead to another painful sexual encounter.

Expect some milk leakage. Sexual stimulation releases oxytocin, the hormone that causes your milk ejection, or letdown, reflex. Your breasts might leak when you make love and even spray your partner in the face when you orgasm. If that's a problem (and who says it has to be?), nurse your baby before you have sex or wear a bra and nursing pads. In any case, you'll want to keep a towel handy. Those things are loaded and they might just go off!

Take your time. It's been a while, but a new mom's body is too sensitive to rush things. Dad, you've waited this long, a few more minutes won't hurt. Foreplay should be long and relaxed.

Guys, don't feel that you absolutely have to finish what you've started. If you're at home, your baby might cry right in the middle of the event you've waited so patiently for. It's not anybody's fault. This is one of those times when you have to switch gears from "lover" to "father" so fast you might feel like you've left your transmission lying somewhere along the road. If you want to score a few points toward the next time, go get the baby and bring her to your wife to nurse.

Golden Opportunities

Once you've broken the ice that first time, you'll need to find more time for romance in the future. It might sound like Mission Impossible, but you can plan for those special times with your partner. Just stay as well rested as you can and keep track of the times during the day and night when your baby is blissfully asleep. Those are your opportunities!

It can take anywhere from a few weeks to an entire year for sex to become as comfortable as it was before pregnancy. Then you'll face a whole new set of challenges. Your child is mobile. If you make love when she's awake, she will find you: They're like bloodhounds.

It's absolutely vital that you not leave your toddler unattended for more than a minute or two. If you must be away from her, remove any hazards from the room and take along the baby monitor. It only takes moments for tragedy to strike an active child.

Once again, it's time to get creative. You've got to take the opportunity for sex when you can get it. If your child loves a certain TV show, that might be your chance. Although you might dislike him now, you may one day be grateful for Barney the Dinosaur.

Even after your toddler has settled into a big-kid bed, you're not safe. Toddlers still tend to walk right in on you in the middle of things, so keep the bedroom door closed, but don't lock it. It won't help. There's nothing like your child yelling for mommy outside the door to put an end to the mood. Just be ready to assume a casual position and have a plausible story prepared for when you're caught.

Your Body

The weeks and months following the birth of your baby are a time of transition for your body. Internally, your uterus, cervix, and vagina are recovering. Breastfeeding helps. When your baby nurses, you will feel your uterus contract. At first, it can hurt, but after the uterus regains its normal size, those contractions often become pleasurable.

FACTS

Kegel exercises are a great way to firm up the muscles in the pelvic floor. Do them as often as you can. To make sure you're doing it right, occasionally practice while you're urinating.

1. Tense up your vaginal and anal muscles as if you were trying to stop a stream of urine.
2. Hold the tension for five seconds.
3. Relax and repeat three to five times.

Like your uterus, your vagina was stretched by childbirth. Many women worry that their vaginas will never regain their predelivery size and wonder if their husbands will find sex less satisfying than before. However, the vagina is a truly remarkable organ. It can expand to accommodate a baby's head and then shrink back to its normal size in just a few days. If you want to accelerate the process along, just tighten your pelvic muscles. Kegel exercises are very effective.

Men, you might really enjoy some of the changes in your wife's body. Remember, there's only one right answer to the question "How do I look?" That answer is "Beautiful." Disparaging comments about your mate's body, even in jest, can destroy the intimacy your relationship needs to last the test of time. A mother's body isn't the body of a girl. It's a woman's body. It's fuller, softer, and more sensuous.

On the other hand, don't go overboard praising your lover's new looks. For example, if you enjoy her somewhat-enhanced cleavage too much, she'll come to believe that her nonlactating breasts are less desirable.

Fertility and Milk Production

Breastfeeding is nature's own form of birth control. If you exclusively breastfeed your baby, you might find that no other contraceptive is necessary. A drop in estrogen production is one of the hormonal changes necessary for milk production to begin and that results in reduced fertility. Doctors call it lactational amenorrhea. Your menstrual cycle stops. Your fertility is so drastically cut that it's like you're using the pill. For a woman with lactational amenorrhea, there's less than a 2 percent chance of conception.

Despite this remarkable contraceptive power, most authorities advise women to use an additional form of birth control to be safe. The reason behind this recommendation is simple. Lactational amenorrhea is easily interrupted, and you might ovulate before the return of your menses. Some women are simply caught off guard.

With precautions, lactational amenorrhea can last at least six months. Some mothers maintain it for much longer. If you plan to rely on breastfeeding as your contraception, here are some guidelines.

Breastfeed exclusively. Do not supplement with any formula or food, or even a bottle of human milk, for at least the first six months.

Don't use pacifiers or bottles. Pacify your baby at your breast only.

Stay as close to your baby as possible. Every woman is different. Some women will begin ovulating again if they are separated from their child for as little as three or four hours. Consider sleeping with your baby or at least close by in the same room.

Nurse your older baby often. Your baby should breastfeed at least eight times in a twenty-four-hour period. Feed at least every six hours, and keep your total daily suckling time to a minimum of sixty minutes.

When your menses returns or your baby reaches six months of age, the reliability of this natural contraceptive is reduced and you should immediately begin using another form of birth control.

Birth Control

If you feel the need to use contraception, you need to be aware of the impact other methods might have on your breastfeeding experience and, possibly, your baby. The safest choice while nursing is a method that doesn't involve chemicals. That means natural family planning, condoms, diaphragms, and cervical caps. The next best choices are products using spermacides like foams, gels, and sponges.

Avoid contraceptive pills that are high in estrogen. They can reduce your milk production. The more common progestin-only pills are considered safe for breastfeeding mothers, as are progestin injections or subdermal implants. For breastfeeding women, injections like Depo-Provera are slightly less effective than implants like Norplant. Although hormonal steroids have not been shown to pose any risk to your baby, they do pass into your milk in small amounts. Some health care professionals worry about early exposure of infants to these compounds and advise breastfeeding mothers to delay their use.

Talk to your doctor for more information about birth control options.

CHAPTER 18

Siblings and Family Life

I magine this: One day your husband arrives home with another woman. "Honey, I love you so much, I wanted another one just like you. I will be spending most of my time with her, but you'll grow to love her and she'll be a great addition to our family." Now imagine what a child would feel if you brought a new baby home without taking steps to help her prepare emotionally.

Family Transitions

New babies are big adjustments, and children experience a wide variety of reactions based on their age and maturity levels. There may be some regression, like bed-wetting or loss of interest in potty training. Toddlers might want to taste breastmilk or suck on a bottle, even after they've been weaned from both. There might be feelings of excitement, anger, or sadness, often all three.

It takes time for feelings to surface, and young children often don't have the words to express them once they do. Sometimes the feelings are just too big for words. All of these reactions are normal and the best way to deal with them is to prepare well in advance.

Toddlers (One to Three)

Toddlers are busy, independent, mobile, curious, active, and often oblivious to the fact that a new baby is in the house, unless it somehow affects their agenda or their possessions. Most parents of toddlers know Toddler Property Laws by now: "What's mine is mine and what's yours is mine, unless it's broken, then it's yours but all the small chokable pieces are still mine."

QUESTIONS?

What are common regressive behaviors in toddlers?
Clinging, whining, crying, bed-wetting, and night waking are common regressive behaviors. All of these reactions are normal but patience will see you through. Children should not be punished or rewarded for regressive behavior. Ignore those things you can and be patient with the rest.

Toddler Property Laws apply to you, too. You belong to your toddler, and there will be some level of jealousy with limited lap time and attention. Your toddler is used to being the baby and to being treated as such. The shift from "baby" to "big brother or sister" is a change of status that can leave your toddler feeling displaced.

Make arrangements for your toddler to stay with a nurturing adult while you're in the hospital. Toddlers have difficulty with abrupt transitions and often suffer from separation anxiety. It's best to prepare early and to make their stay sound like an adventure. Once you're admitted to the hospital, make frequent phone calls to check on her. She needs to hear your voice and know that you'll come back soon. Don't forget to pack her lovies, like a favorite blanket or stuffed animal. These are useful transitional objects that keep her connected to you while you're physically apart.

Sexual Education

You've entered the "why" stage of parenting. When answering toddler questions, it's important to keep your answers simple, short, age-appropriate, and honest. It's easy to overload a toddler who wants only his specific question answered. Others will follow, to be certain, and you might be answering the same question in several different, yet creative, ways. Always focus on one question at one time.

Your toddler may take an interest in breastfeeding, too. After the birth of her baby brother, four-year-old Jennifer asked her mother, Linda, if she could have a taste of her breastmilk. Linda allowed it, and Jennifer never asked again. When Suzanne nursed Ian, Meaghan would grab her doll, lift her shirt, and "nurse" her baby. These are important lessons in both nutrition and nurturing, as well as positive female role modeling. Young girls turn into grown-up women, and they need to know the rules of the game.

Toolbox Tricks

Toddlers benefit from learning about babies by observing them in action. Before your baby is born, invite friends with infants to visit so your toddler can explore and learn about gentle touch. Toddlers continue to learn best through sensory contact, so touch, taste, sight, smell, and hearing are important teaching strategies to use.

When your baby arrives home, explore her together. Count fingers and toes. Touch her skin. Allow your toddler to hold the baby with supervision.

When it's time to nurse, have a basket full of toys, books, crayons, envelopes, stickers, old checkbooks, paper, and interesting household items handy. Pull it out only when you breastfeed, so it gives the basket special meaning. Have snacks ready, too. Children will often wait until your newborn has latched on perfectly and is nursing contentedly to ask for a drink or a snack. If you keep nutritious snacks and juice boxes in your basket, they'll be ready when you need them.

ESSENTIALS

Like the rest of us, toddlers have good and not-so-good days. Accept these feelings and remember that they are often short-lived. Parents of toddlers know that mood dictates behavior. Anticipate when they'll need a nap or a snack, and meet their needs before major meltdowns occur.

If you have a sling, you can nurse your newborn as you take your toddler for a walk around the block. With time, you'll learn how to nurse one-handed. You can use the other hand to hold your toddler or help turn the pages of his storybook.

Preschoolers (Three to Five)

It's difficult to predict how your preschooler will react to your new baby. When visiting you and your new addition in the hospital, most preschoolers will take little interest in the baby and will be more curious about how high the hospital bed can go or whether they can keep the bendy straws in the Styrofoam cup.

Don't expect immediate bonding between siblings, and don't be surprised if there's a complete lack of interest from your child. It doesn't mean jealousy. As new parents, we're on guard to protect our children from feeling emotions we label as negative, but having those feelings are an important part of growing up.

Sexual Education

Preschoolers have a natural curiosity about their bodies and those of their friends. This is the "doctor" stage of development. Preschoolers can identify themselves and their peers as girls or boys and are entering a sexual identity stage. They explore their bodies enthusiastically and know what makes them feel good. Pregnancy and birth are excellent times to begin light sexual education with your preschooler. Again, answers should be short and sweet. Give real names to body parts and refer to your breasts as "breasts" and not "babas."

Three-year-olds are often fascinated by the diaper change of an opposite-gendered baby. This experience provides golden opportunities to talk about body parts and sexual differences in a healthy way. Defining sexual organs by their appropriate names sets the stage for healthy sexual identity now and later in life.

Toolbox Tricks

Preschoolers love books. A trip to the library to gather books about newborn care is a helpful way to introduce your new baby. Choose books with lots of photographs.

FACTS

Preschoolers often experience regressive behaviors just like toddlers. You might notice more baby talk, potty accidents, and some dependency issues. After all, they notice how much attention the new baby gets from these same behaviors. These regressions are normal and will disappear with time.

Preschoolers also love art, as well, and will create "elaborate" drawings of a circle head and stick legs to represent a person. More advanced artists might include stick arms and eyeballs, but that's usually only on request. You can extend a drawing session while you're nursing by asking your preschooler to add facial features, clothing, accessories, action, and background. A basket of colored pencils, crayons, blank paper, notebooks, and coloring books should hold their interest for the length of a feeding session.

Teach your preschooler the art of hand massage. Make this her important job with the new baby. Let her know you appreciate her help in the caregiving role.

Ask your preschooler to share stories about her new brother or sister. Those stories are often heavily veiled discussions about their own feelings and private thoughts. Help them give words and meaning to their feelings.

How can I be sure my preschooler has enough time with children his own age?
Schedule play dates with other children or enroll in a half-day early education program. Socialization with same-aged peers is important for your preschooler and gives you special time alone with your newborn.

School-Aged Children (Six to Twelve)

School-aged children are often enthusiastic and excited about having a new baby in the house. They are busy with school, friends, and outside activities and often view a new baby as a novelty.

Older children approach babies playfully. They model parenting skills, too. It's sometimes like watching a reflection of yourself as they coo and cuddle with their new infant. Be proud that you've taught them well.

School-aged kids are good at discussing their feelings, especially around bedtime, so make your routines with them sacred. There is something magical about the bedtime hour that makes kids open up. It's dim and intimate, and communication flows. It might simply be that your kids don't want to go to sleep, but regardless of your child's motivation, take advantage of these opportunities by sharing feelings. Listen with an open mind and an open heart.

Sexual Education

This is the stage where kids think kissing is icky. This is also about the time we ran across those National Geographic photos of bare-breasted women when we were kids. It is an excellent time to have a discussion about the birds and the bees, if your child is interested and you're comfortable with the topic. As with children of any age, it's important not to overload them with information. It might be helpful finding out what they already know and building on that.

Breastfeeding gives chidren a healthy view of the human body. It also demonstrates the natural use of the breast. Children who grow up in breastfeeding homes are often more comfortable about their own bodies and sexual identities than those who don't.

Kids on the school playground are like a fourth-grade secret society. They've shared secrets about how babies are made, as well as dispelled myths about the tooth fairy and other mystical gift-givers. However, there is a lot of misinformation out there. Kids who don't know all the answers often speculate and fill in the blanks with something shocking or downright hilarious.

Toolbox Tricks

Ask your school-aged child to write a letter to the new baby welcoming her home. Take a picture of your new baby so Dad can pack it in the lunch box as a surprise. Because breastfed babies are extremely mobile, ask your child if he would like you to bring the baby to kindergarten show-and-tell.

School-aged children still need to spend quality time with you. Make arrangements for Dad to stay with smaller children as you and your third grader go out for ice cream. Ask your child to plan a special one-on-one activity for an afternoon out.

School-aged kids are great entertainers! Have them try these games with your new baby to make her laugh: hold a silly face contest, play tickle games, recite "This Little Piggy," play peek-a-boo, play puppets, make animal sounds, or blow bubbles. Involve the whole family in entertainment!

Preserve routines as much as possible. Children need stability, security, and the ability to predict the day's events. They also need a good night's sleep and healthy snacks and meals. Too many changes too fast can leave everyone in a tailspin. Patience and planned transition time will help smooth the way for major changes in your family's life.

Teenagers (Thirteen and Over)

Eeewwww. Enough said? You had sex, and your teenager is mortified that someone your age still engages in such activities. On top of that, you're breastfeeding. You've bared your breasts in front of other people when your teen thinks you should be hiding in a closet. Teenagers might not be used to seeing breasts (other than a quick glance at their own) outside of PG-13 movies. In addition, their own emerging sexuality makes it difficult to think about their parents in sexual terms.

Teens have entered a very dramatic period in their lives. Their hor-mones play an important role in their behavior. They are often emotional, easily embarrassed, moody, withdrawn, and private. They're working on acquiring grown-up skills while coming to terms with their own changing bodies. Sometimes their bodies are maturing faster than they are.

Sexual Education

Pregnancy and breastfeeding are excellent lessons in human development. During the teen years, much misinformation is shared on the telephone or through the rumor mill. These are big gossip years.

Having a baby in the house can be a wonderful lesson about birth control. While many high school home economics classes require teens to lug around five-pound bags of flour for weeks to teach about family planning, teens with new babies in their homes should be exempt. They often have firsthand experience with their new sibling. Learning the responsibilities of infant care firsthand can frighten many teenagers away from early sexual encounters out of fear of pregnancy, or at the very least, can encourage the use of reliable birth control.

Observing a parent breastfeeding an infant teaches important information about the function of the breast in relation to infant nutrition. It also demonstrates bonding in action. Children learn a lot about relationships by watching their parents.

Toolbox Tricks

Teens do a lot of journaling and diary writing. If you have difficulty communicating verbally with your teen, write him a letter or send him an e-mail. Kids need to know that they are valued and appreciated. Teens, like all children, need security and stability, particularly now, when fears of school failure, the future, and opposite-gendered relationships are first on their minds. Communicate and spend time with your teenager as best you can.

Teamwork

Pick a good time to discuss with your partner what needs to be done. Agree that your home doesn't need to be spotless. The sooner you get used to some degree of disorganization, the easier it is to be a parent. Children naturally make messes. It's part of life and part of learning, so don't stress out over little things that aren't really so important in the long run.

Adjusting to life with a new baby is not the time to fixate on the things that should be done, or should be done differently. You need to concentrate on breastfeeding and caring for your infant. Provide constructive direction to your helpers, and remember that they're still learning, too.

Sometimes, it's hard for mothers to let their mates care for the baby. Remember, your husband doesn't need to interact with your child in the same way you do in order to be a good parent. Each of us has his or her own style, and these styles are all valid as long as they support the safety and healthy development of our children.

Toddlers are big helpers, too. They love to help with housework and model your behaviors. Give them a mismatched mitten and let them dust the low spots under tables and around the living room. Be sensitive about what they are able to do developmentally and what they are willing to do based on their mood.

Preschoolers often seek ways to assist you before you even ask. They often mimic parents in the roles they play and have rich imaginations. A well-meaning four-year-old might make you a breakfast of raw carrots with maple syrup to show you that he cares. Young children are helpful at this stage, and are usually willing to fetch diapers and wipes. They might even ask to change the diaper themselves. Preschoolers can sing and entertain your newborn, tell her made-up stories, and recite nursery rhymes.

School-aged kids are a huge help around the house. They usually have their chore lists by now, like feeding the pets, cleaning their rooms, or folding their own laundry. You can now slowly increase these chores. Children this age are enthusiastic about diapering, holding, rocking, and singing lullabies. They can take pictures for the family photo album, offer a bottle of expressed milk, bathe the baby with adult supervision, and safety-proof the living room.

Teens can offer paid baby-sitting services, entertainment, and increased household responsibility.

The adjustment to new babies is what makes families families. Children learn important life lessons through this experience. Compromise, negotiation, kindness, sharing, trading, humor, cooperation, and frustration are all important to survive and be happy in the world.

The Family Pet

To prepare your pet for the arrival of your baby, have Dad bring your infant's unwashed blanket or cap home on the night before your baby comes home. Allow your pet to have plenty of time exploring her scent.

Before your pet greets your baby, it's important for you to greet him. If you've both been away for a couple of days, your pet will be excited to see you. Greet him first, then while sitting on the couch, allow him to gently greet your new addition. Introducing your family pet to the new baby should be a slow and gentle process. Your pet will learn to recognize and identify your baby through scent, so he will spend a lot of time sniffing (and perhaps sneezing) to commit her smell to memory.

The best pets for small children are those that are gentle, confident, affectionate, loyal, intelligent, patient, sociable, trustworthy, and reliable. Even lazy pets are good for babies. Cats in general are good choices.

FACTS

The best dog breeds for small children include: Labrador retrievers, bulldogs, hound dogs, boxers, setters, Great Danes, Newfoundlands, Saint Bernards, sheep dogs, collies, beagles, and spaniels. Any dogs that are not completely domesticated are poor choices and should be avoided.

As a rule, bigger dogs do very well with young children and smaller dogs do not. Some dogs are high-strung, wiry, anxious, emotionally disturbed, or have special needs. These conditions affect their behavior as well as their adaptability to your new baby. Infants develop into curious toddlers, so your pet should be one that children can grow into.

A dog's temperament is inherited but can be changed by both the events in his life and training. It's a unique balance of nature and nurture. Some breeds are friendlier, smarter, more tolerant and patient than others. These dogs are also more easily trained.

CHAPTER 19

How Long Should I Breastfeed?

You are successfully breastfeeding your baby and everything seems to be going great. Eventually though, you'll begin to wonder, "How long should I breastfeed?" Everyone seems to have an opinion on this one, and most will share it. Some folks will warn you against "coddling" older infants and toddlers. Others might think it's "inappropriate" to nurse a child beyond a particular age. In the end, the decision is yours.

Physical Limits

How many years can you breastfeed? The short answer is: all of them. Women are generally able to nurse their children as long as they need to. If milk is being taken from the breast, more milk will be produced to take its place. From puberty to death you can produce milk. Yes, that long. Menopause is no obstacle.

There's also no physical limit on the age of your nursing child. Although breastmilk is all your baby needs for the first six months of life, older children continue to get immunities and vitamins from your milk for as long as you let them.

Now, just because you can nurse forever doesn't mean you will. Even if you don't actively stop your child from breastfeeding, she will probably stop on her own. If left to the child, breastfeeding usually comes to a natural conclusion by the time they reach three to four years of age. Of course, you can stop long before then if you decide you want to.

Medical Recommendations

We've established that you could breastfeed your child for years. The real question is, "How long should I breastfeed?" not "How long can I breastfeed?" There are quite a few recommendations from the medical community and, luckily, they all agree.

The AAP suggests that all babies should breastfeed exclusively for their first six months, and as long after that as the family chooses.

The ILCA believes that all mothers should nurse exclusively for a minimum of six months, then add other foods and continue to nurse until two years or as long as they can.

The U.N.'s WHO endorses breastfeeding with no other foods for at least the child's first six months of life. In an April 2001 Note to the Press, however, The WHO ". . . recognizes that some mothers will be unable to, or choose not to, follow this recommendation."

In short, the medical community says you should breastfeed exclusively for at least your baby's first six months of life. Doctors and researchers recognize the value of breastfeeding with no other supplemental foods for the baby during that first half-year. They also recognize the benefits of continued breastfeeding along with other foods until your baby's second birthday and beyond.

Any time spent breastfeeding your child is better than no time at all. The first few weeks of your baby's life are some of the most critical for his health. Your breastmilk plays a vital role during this time, and your baby's immune system needs the boost.

So, the simple answer is this: You should nurse your baby for at least the first six months, and continue for as long afterward as both you and your baby want.

Cultural and Historical Issues

Many of the truths we hold as absolute are nothing more than the traditions in which we've been raised. Although some of these traditions are valuable, the ones that interfere with breastfeeding harm children and their families, and modern American culture is not as breastfeeding-friendly as many others around the world are.

In the first part of our country's history, breastfeeding was as American as apple pie. From colonization through the nineteenth century, 95 percent of American children were breastfed for two to four years. However, by the 1950s, 1960s, and early 1970s, breastfeeding was becoming increasingly rare. Bottle feeding of infant formula was considered more proper and sophisticated by one set of American women, and liberating from traditional roles by another set.

Today, we're lucky. The pendulum of public opinion has swung back in favor of breastfeeding. Accompanying practices like public nursing, which Americans once considered "primitive" or "unladylike," are becoming increasingly accepted, even unremarkable. At the same time, the increase in popularity that breastfeeding has enjoyed over the past twenty-five years has raised a new generation that's more supportive of lactation.

Nursing by the Numbers

More and more families are enjoying the benefits of breastfeeding, but the numbers remain lower than health care professionals would like to see.

In 1995, only 60 percent of mothers in the United States were breastfeeding at discharge from the hospital following childbirth. Unfortunately, just 22 percent were still breastfeeding six months later, and a mere 2 percent nursed their child beyond one year of age.

The United States is unusual in this respect, since the average age for complete weaning from the breast worldwide is about four years. Many people feel that the availability of a wide range of nutritious foods makes breastfeeding beyond a year unnecessary, even emotionally harmful, but there is no evidence to support either conclusion. To the contrary, research clearly shows that children benefit from breastmilk until at least their third or fourth birthdays.

ESSENTIALS

Some people will criticize your decision to breastfeed beyond your baby's first few months. Tell the critic your doctor's recommendations. You might even explain the benefits of nursing. To people who say, "You're still nursing that child?" just smile and tell them, "Yes. And thanks for noticing!"

Despite the many benefits of extending breastfeeding beyond a year, American popular culture seems resistant to the idea. There have even been charges brought against women for nursing school-aged children. No convictions have resulted, but an irrational discomfort with extended nursing is apparent.

Critics of extended breastfeeding believe that it fosters dependence and immaturity. However, growth is a process that can't be rushed. Stability, love, and security are the foundations of healthy growth. Breastfeeding helps a mother nurture her child's development.

Professional Opinions

Pushing our children to wean before they're ready might actually result in insecurities and bad habits. But most Americans do it anyway. As a result, older toddlers fight to keep their pacifiers and children entering kindergarten still suck their thumbs. The need to suck can't be extinguished by forced weaning.

The AAP puts the blame on a widespread lack of societal support for breastfeeding. Specifically, the AAP points to:

- Apathetic and misinformed doctors
- Insufficient breastfeeding education
- Counterproductive hospital policies
- Unnecessary interruption of breastfeeding
- Premature discharge from the hospital
- Shortage of routine follow-up care and home health care
- Maternal employment
- Popular media depiction of bottle feeding
- Advertising and promotion of infant formula

Many researchers would add at least three other items to that list.

Preoccupation with the sexuality of the breast. American culture regards breasts as such inherently sexual organs, that their primary function is sometimes threatened. We can't show photos of breastfeeding on billboards for fear of offending someone, so babies with bottles smile out at us from every ad. Even women who breastfeed are often uncomfortable with the idea of nursing a toddler or a preschooler.

Preference for scientific or technological solutions. Bottles and formula strike Americans as more scientific than breastfeeding. Western tradition relies heavily on technology, and it's generally paid off for us. However, we've developed an almost religious faith in science and an unhealthy acceptance of infant formula has resulted. We're too quick to assume that a few decades of study can duplicate millions of years of natural selection.

Consumer culture. We are a nation of consumers, serviced by a huge commercial industry. Breastfeeding just doesn't give us as much to buy as bottle feeding of infant formula does. Corporations push artificial feeding in advertisements and promotions. Manufacturers provide free samples to hospitals and doctors, knowing that an unsure new mom might just decide to use some formula since she has it. After the resulting nipple confusion and decreased milk production, the continued sale of formula is assured.

FACTS

Women who continue to nurse older children—and there are thousands of them—often keep out of the public eye. No one wants to feel like an outcast because of the way she chooses to care for her child.

Many of us grew up with baby bottles and infant formula. We used them ourselves and saw them on TV and in magazines. For most Americans, bottles and formula seem more normal than breastfeeding. However, nature's not a democracy. We can't change what's healthiest for our children by popular practice.

Toddler Nursing

In the United States, mothers who practice extended nursing breastfeed their child an average of 2.75 years. Why nurse a toddler? The benefits of breastfeeding a toddler are the same as they are for younger children.

- Breastmilk continues to be a wonderful source of nutrition, regardless of anything else your child eats.
- Antibodies in your milk continue to protect your toddler, even if he nurses just once a day.
- Breastfeeding comforts children.
- Toddler nursing might be the only snuggle time you get with your busy child while he's awake.

- Breastmilk can be tolerated by sick children who are unable to stomach other foods.

The more you meet your child's needs, the more independent and confident she will grow. Knowing that you're there for her as she continues to explore gives her the courage to take on a huge, exciting unknown world. Every successful mission will bolster her confidence and increase her sense of independence. Breastfeeding helps.

Styles and Tips

Nursing a toddler presents some unique challenges, but they're usually no problem if you know how to deal with them in advance.

First, how will your child let you know when he wants to nurse? A one-year-old who announces that he wants "boobies" might be cute around the house, but when he says the same thing in public it can leave you glowing red with embarrassment. This is a problem you can prevent by choosing a good code word for breastfeeding early in your relationship. "Nurse" is a good one, but anything you like will work.

QUESTIONS?

What do you do with toddler's roaming hands?
Hold your child's hand and kiss his little fingers or keep a special toy or book nearby that he can hold only while nursing. A textured rattle is sometimes a good choice. The name of the game is distraction.

If you master the name change, your next hurdle will be explaining that you won't be feeding in public so much anymore. With such a general misunderstanding of toddler nursing in America, public feedings can leave you feeling humiliated by the stares and whispers of uninformed strangers. Your child is probably used to nursing whenever he wants. Any new restrictions are bound to evoke a tantrum in a headstrong toddler, so be ready for it. This is a good time to begin explaining the difference between "public" and "private." Or you might choose to confidently nurse in public knowing that you are doing the best for your child.

Toddlers like to move. They've only recently mastered walking, running, and climbing, and they love to find new ways to use their bodies. Unfortunately, constant motion and breastfeeding don't go well together. Your little gymnast might decide at some point that nursing would be more fun if he could twist, turn, and climb all over you while suckling away. Ouch! Some kids go from standing to hanging upside down over your shoulder in a single feeding session.

ESSENTIALS

As a child spends less time feeding at his mother's breast, he can spend more time with Dad. This is a great opportunity for early literacy! Dad's lap can be a great refuge to cuddle and read a good book.

If your child's acrobatics are more than you can take, the best solution is to end the breastfeeding session. Don't get angry, but rather announce firmly but gently that nursing time (or whatever you two call it) is a time to lie still. This is the same kind of strategy used to stop nipple biting, and it's usually effective after a very short while.

Your Child's Individual Needs

You are an island of security for your toddler in an unexplored world. Your little adventurer will travel away from you for ever-increasing amounts of time and distance, but he needs to know he can return for protection, comfort, and anything else he needs. He's also eager to share what he's experienced with you and let you help him understand it.

It's important that you treat your child as an individual. At the same time, pay attention to your own feelings. You're the mother, and you know what's best for your particular child. If you go at the pace that's right for both you and your child, you can continue to enjoy the breastfeeding experience.

Nursing Through Pregnancy

If you're breastfeeding your toddler or older child when you become pregnant, you might be thinking about weaning. However, pregnancy and lactation are more compatible than once believed, and continued breastfeeding helps an older child feel secure during this time of change.

Obstetricians once routinely advised pregnant women to discontinue breastfeeding for fear of a miscarriage. Nipple stimulation caused by suckling releases oxytocin in your body. This hormone causes a number of things to occur, including milk ejection (letdown) and uterine contractions.

Although oxytocin is released in a pregnant mother's body when she nurses her child, the uterine tissues are less receptive to its effects than they would be if she weren't lactating. Current research seems to indicate that this decreased sensitivity to oxytocin stays strong throughout the first four months of pregnancy. Even after that time, you can continue to nurse your older child with confidence as long as everything else about your pregnancy is normal.

If you have a history of miscarriages, are diagnosed as "at risk" for early labor, or notice strong contractions while breastfeeding, you should stop nursing your child. Contact your doctor immediately. You might be advised to discontinue any nipple stimulation, including sex.

Throughout your pregnancy, you and your toddler will have to accommodate some changes. Beginning in about the fourth month, your breastmilk will decrease in volume and begin to change into the colostrum your newborn needs. Your toddler might or might not give any notice to these changes. Some little ones continue right along, nursing like normal. Others will decide that your milk tastes funny and they'll nurse less frequently.

If you decide to stop breastfeeding, even for a day, it's important for you to find other ways to bond with your toddler. This is also a great opportunity for Dad to spend a little more time with his child. Both parents can read, snuggle, and play more with their toddler whenever breastfeeding is interrupted. These other activities will keep him happy and secure in the knowledge that he's not being replaced. With all of the attention the new baby gets, it's common for your older child to feel left out.

Tandem Nursing

Tandem nursing is when you breastfeed two or more children at the same time. It's a great way to keep older children connected with Mom and teach the value of sharing.

The term tandem nursing is really a misnomer. Most mothers who breastfeed both a newborn and an older child don't do it simultaneously. Usually, the newborn nurses first, and then Mom is available to breastfeed the older child. While common, this approach is not without its drawbacks.

ESSENTIALS

In the first few days of your newborn's life, let him nurse first and nurse as often as he wants. This system of feeding is important to ensure that he receives all the colostrum he needs.

Like serial nursing of twins and triplets, a mother who feeds her toddler after her newborn might feel like all she does is breastfeed. That can make the process feel less like bonding, and more like an assembly line. Even if you don't mind the arrangement, your toddler might. Depending on how you handled his feedings through your latest pregnancy, your toddler might feel suddenly displaced.

For some moms, simultaneous breastfeeding is the solution. With a child on each breast, nursing takes a lot less time. There's no perceived favorite and both children stay close to Mom. They might even bond with each other more effectively as they share the satisfaction of nursing. If you find that you don't like it, then try something else. There is no right or wrong answer here. The goal is to find a way to keep all of you happy. Ideally, tandem nursing should be a win-win-win situation.

CHAPTER 20

Infant Nutrition and Introducing Solids

The move to solids is a great time for Dad to get involved in feeding his baby! The first few months of solid food for your baby are good, messy fun. Your baby will love some foods and respond with smiles and squeals. Other foods will make her look at you with expressions of disgust that seem to say, "What is this horrible stuff you're putting in my mouth?"

First Feedings

Infants have an inborn tongue-thrust reflex. They'll push both the spoon and any food on it out of their mouth. This reflex might have evolved to prevent choking, and it continues to be strong until around six months of age. When it comes to infant feeding, most of what goes in will also come out, one end or the other. Grab your camera, as this will be a perfect Kodak moment. Your baby will wear more food than he eats. You'll want to capture the surprised look on his face when he tries a new taste for the first time. Don't worry that he's not getting enough to eat. More than half of his daily calories will continue to be in the form of human milk or formula.

WHEN IS BABY READY FOR SOLIDS?

There are some general rules of thumb for assessing whether your baby is prepared for a change in diet. If your baby meets these criteria, he's ready for baby food. Use this checklist to help you assess readiness:

❑ Baby is between four and six months of age.

❑ Baby has doubled his birthweight.

❑ Baby can hold his head upright on his own and turn head from side to side.

❑ Baby can sit up assisted or on his own.

❑ Baby shows an interest in what you're eating and wants some, too.

❑ Baby can communicate when he is full.

❑ Baby is still hungry after a daily total thirty-two ounces of breastmilk or formula.

With time, your baby will learn to swallow solids. Babies swallow differently from a bottle, from a cup, and from a straw. They also swallow differently with food. A baby has to take food to the roof of his mouth and squish it. Expect your baby to gag or cough the first couple of times. As he develops better tongue control, he will quickly learn to swallow without sputtering.

You can tell your baby is full if he turns his head away from the food source, closes or clenches his mouth, spits out food, or acts fussy. These are your cues to end the feeding session.

Follow his first few feedings with breastmilk or formula. As your baby grows, you can offer a cup of water or expressed milk to help wash his food down.

FACTS

A word about portions: Your baby's stomach is the size of his tiny fist, just as your stomach is the size of your grown-up fist. If he eats a tablespoon of cereal followed by a full feeding of breastmilk, he will be satisfied. We often overestimate how much children can eat. Use the "rule of fist" as your lifelong guide.

The best time to feed will be when you are relaxed and have time to enjoy each other. Babies take a long time to experience food. They savor new flavors and love new textures. Because babies explore the world through sensory play, don't be surprised if sweet potatoes soon become hair gel. It's a messy process, but a necessary one. Your baby is learning an important new skill, how to eat!

Supplies

Your baby will need some new supplies as he moves into solid foods. You can finally break out all those cute baby bibs he received as shower gifts! Plastic place mats strategically positioned around the room will catch the leaks from thrown sippy cups and long-distance spills. Or you can purchase a large splat mat to put under the highchair. Even the family pet can pitch in.

A plastic or rubber-coated spoon is nice and won't poke your baby's eye out when he tries to use it by himself. You might consider letting him play with the spoon a few days prior to starting solids so he can become familiar with it. Chewing on a coated spoon also helps when your baby's gums are sensitive from teething. A divided plastic dish with high sides is perfect for feeding several different foods at one time, like fruits, vegetables, and cereal. If the plate has suction cups to adhere it to the highchair tray, all the better.

Food Allergies

Although food allergies are pretty rare, they do occur. The foods that are most likely to cause allergies include: peanut products, strawberries, milk products, citrus fruits, tomatoes, egg whites, fish, spinach, and wheat. Wait until your baby is at least a year old to share these foods with her.

Keep a notebook to record your baby's reactions to new foods. If your baby experiences rash, excessive phlegm, coughing, wheezing, watery eyes, diarrhea, vomiting, hives, or any respiratory ailment after the introduction of a new food, contact your pediatrician.

Food Schedules

Foods should be introduced slowly and one at a time. Allow at least three days between introductions so you can identify potential problems. If you have a family history of food allergies, pay special attention to your baby's reactions to new foods.

Cereals

Because babies' digestive systems are still immature, they need foods that are easily absorbed. Iron-fortified infant cereals should be the first foods following breastmilk or formula that baby will experience.

Start with a box of dry rice cereal. Boxes are better bargains than jars, and dry cereals allow you to add human milk or formula. Rice has the fewest allergy-related reactions. Wait at least a week between introducing new cereals. Rice should be followed by oatmeal, then barley. Wheat and mixed cereals can cause allergic reactions in infants younger than one year of age, so it's better to wait on those.

Juice

Juice can be introduced around six to eight months of age. Start with 100 percent grape juice, as this is easiest to digest. Apple and pear juices, although milder than other fruit juices, contain sorbital, a natural fruit sugar our intestines cannot absorb. It ferments in the intestines and causes tummy aches and diarrhea. Grape juice does not contain sorbital. Acidic juices like cranberry, orange, and grapefruit should be delayed until after your baby's first birthday.

In the case of juice, more is not better. It can cause rapid tooth decay because of its high sugar content. It's important that it be fed only in a cup and that a regular toothbrushing routine be established. Juice can also cause obesity and digestive problems, so its use should be limited.

Choose only 100 percent fruit juices. Some doctors recommend that juice be diluted to half-strength, but the WIC program does not. Avoid cans or bottles labeled "juice drink." These have only a small amount of juice added. The first ingredient listed is the main ingredient. Learning to read labels now will help you to make healthy choices as your child grows.

From six to twelve months of age, only four ounces of juice is recommended per day. You can serve small amounts throughout the day or offer one full cup at a sitting. Juice will curb your baby's appetite, so offer it as a snack between meals. As baby gets older, whole unprocessed fruits are a better choice than juice.

Vegetables

Join the "vegetables first" crowd. Babies already have a preference for sweets, so fruits will be readily accepted. Some vegetables, on the other hand, might take some getting used to. Your baby might refuse to eat vegetables if fruits are introduced first.

Baby vegetables come pureed or strained. They have the consistency of applesauce, but not necessarily the texture. Some manufacturers add modified tapioca food starch as a filler to smooth the texture, but this has little or no nutritional value.

Vegetables can be introduced around six months of age. One to two tablespoons per day is all your baby needs for the next three months. A yellow vegetable at lunch and a green vegetable with dinner will provide a balanced and nutritious diet for your baby.

Spinach, beets, and broccoli cause gas and should be avoided until after twelve months of age. They are also high in naturally occuring nitrates, which reduce your baby's ability to transport oxygen through his blood. Use these foods moderately.

Add one new vegetable per week. Watch for reactions such as allergies or diaper rash.

Fruits

Fruits will be enthusiastically explored and accepted by your baby. Fruits without added sugars are best, so mash peaches canned in their own juice or grate a fresh pear. Sugar has no nutritional value and many foods are naturally sweet.

As with vegetables, one to two tablespoons of fruit per day is all a baby needs for healthy development. Add one new fruit per week. Again, watch for signs of allergic reaction.

There are a few precautions you need to take when serving fruits to your baby. Citrus fruits should be avoided until after your baby's first birthday. Dried fruits are sticky and can cause cavities. Apple slices, as well as other raw fruits and vegetables, can be a choking hazard. When your baby is old enough to tolerate oranges and tangerines, remember to remove the seeds.

Meats

Meats are generally introduced around nine months of age. They are important sources of iron and protein. Instead of buying jarred meats, you can simply save a few tablespoons of the unseasoned meat you're cooking for dinner and mash it for your baby. Making your own ground chicken, pork, beef, or turkey costs less than commercially prepared foods. Serve meats warm but not hot.

Eggs should be cooked and all egg whites removed. Egg whites are a known allergen. Hard-boil an egg and serve the mashed yolk. If your baby develops an allergy to eggs before his first birthday, tell your pediatrician. Egg whites are used as a base in the measles-mumps-rubella vaccine your baby will have when he's fifteen to eighteen months of age. If your child has an egg allergy, the immunization could make him sick.

Breastmilk and Bottles

Some mothers nurse before offering solids to take the edge off of baby's appetite, while others wait to nurse until afterward. Try it both ways. You know your baby best and whatever you choose will be right for him.

It's important to continue breastfeeding as your baby learns to eat solid food. When infants are six months of age or younger, solids are not a substitute for breastmilk. Solids are a supplement to breastfeeding. Your milk contains the nutrients he needs, and because he's still getting the majority of his calories through your milk, nursing should be continued.

Sometimes offering solids can be a battle. Babies may fight spoons, cereals, or juice cups. If, by ten months, your baby absolutely refuses solid food, it's time to contact your pediatrician. There might be a problem with his oral-motor development.

However, older babies tend to breastfeed less and take fewer bottles as they eat more and more solids. This is often the time when most babies decide to self-wean. Weaning is accelerated by introducing new foods to an infant's diet. If you want to preserve the breastfeeding relationship, continue to offer the breast as often as your baby will accept it. If your baby refuses, it may become a battle of wills. It may also be time to make changes in your breastfeeding routine.

RECOMMENDED DAILY ALLOWANCE OF FOOD
FOR INFANTS UNDER ONE YEAR OF AGE

AGE	FOOD	SERVINGS	AMOUNT PER SERVING
0–4 mos.	Breastmilk	8–12	
	Formula	4–8	4–8 oz. (up to 32 oz.)
4–6 mos.	Breastmilk	6–8	
	Formula	4–8	4–8 oz. (up to 32 oz.)
	Iron-Fortified Cereal	2	1–2 tablespoons
6–9 mos.	Breastmilk	5–7	
	Formula	4	8 oz. (up to 32 oz.)
	Iron-Fortified Cereal	2	2–4 tablespoons
	Vegetables	2	2 tablespoons
	Fruits	2	2 tablespoons
	Juice	1	2–4 oz. in a sippy cup
9–12 mos.	Breastmilk	4–5	
	Formula	4	8 oz.
	Iron-Fortified Cereal	2	3–4 tablespoons
	Vegetables	2	3–4 tablespoons
	Fruits	2	3–4 tablespoons
	Juice	1	2–4 oz.
	Bread	2	½ slice
	Crackers		1–2
	Meats	2	3–4 tablespoons

Safe Handling and Storage of Baby Foods

You were careful to ensure clean hands and breasts when you started nursing. Cleanliness is even more important now. You can't always know where food has been or what it's been exposed to.

It's also important to serve baby foods from a dish, not straight from the jar. For smaller infants, you can measure the appropriate amounts in divided containers. Throw away any uneaten food from the dish. Bacteria from baby's mouth will contaminate the food and continue to grow, and that could make your baby sick.

BABY FOOD STORAGE: HOMEMADE OR OPENED JARS		
Food	Refrigerator	Freezer
Fruits	2–3 days	6–8 months
Vegetables	2–3 days	6–8 months
Meats	1 day	1–2 months
Eggs	1 day	1–2 months
Mixed Foods	1–2 days	1–2 months

Finger Foods

Around seven to nine months, offer your child finger foods. Bite-size pieces of unsalted crackers, iron-fortified toast (avoid whole wheat), and Rice Chex or Cheerios are great foods for little mouths and hands. Baby is developing an ability to draw his thumb and fingers together to pick up small items (including the lint under your couch) and bring them to his mouth. His saliva will quickly transform crackers to mush, but whole saltines or broken bits of teething biscuits can be chokable. Keep an eye on all finger foods. Babies will sometimes swallow without chewing, so caution is recommended.

The following foods are extremely chokable and should be avoided until after your baby's first birthday: popcorn, marshmallows, nuts, candy, pretzels, raw vegetables, grapes, hot dogs, peanut butter, peanuts. Babies put almost everything in their mouth. Now is the time to enroll in an infant first aid and CPR class.

Dairy products like cottage or string cheeses and frozen yogurt can be introduced around your baby's first birthday, as can whole, homogenized milk. At this age, babies need less than thirty-two ounces of milk per day. Be sure to use whole milk, not 2 percent, skim, or chocolate. The fat in whole milk is important for brain development. Offer milk in a cup but not in a bottle. The bottle can now be used for water at bedtime. Water will often help your toddler lose interest in the bottle, making it easier to let go.

Toothbrushing

You can begin to clean an infant's gums even before the eruption of her first tooth. A small piece of moist gauze is sufficient. After the first tooth comes in around five to six months of age, you can offer a cool wet washcloth to chew on between and after meals.

After your baby's first birthday, introduce a toddler toothbrush. You can purchase these at any department store. They are smaller than child-sized brushes and have fewer bristles. Use only water to clean teeth, since toddlers will often swallow toothpaste.

Visit a pediatric dentist between the ages of two and three. She will tell you when to begin flossing and will provide additional dental education.

Most importantly, remember to model good dental hygiene and your baby will follow your lead!

CHAPTER 21

Employment, Child Care, and Breastfeeding

Breastfeeding when you return to work can be a challenge. It requires a great deal of commitment and determination to maintain your milk supply and to advocate for yourself and your baby. You need the support of all the players on your team. The assistance of the right child care provider, a supportive employer, and a breastfeeding-friendly workplace can ensure your continued success.

Finding a Breastfeeding-Friendly Day Care

The search for day care often begins before your baby is even born. The best day cares have lengthy waiting lists, and rightly so. In the day care business, you often get what you pay for.

It's especially important to find a provider who shares your parenting philosophies. Make a list of key issues that are important to you and discuss them with each potential caregiver. Be sure to ask questions about their policies and procedures on breastfeeding and the handling and storage of human milk. There are several types of day care environments to consider, from commercial care centers to private, in-home care. Only you know what's best for your baby.

Formal Day Care Centers

Most formal day care centers are licensed facilities that meet state health and safety standards. State officials maintain quality through random observations and inspections. Consider the following pros and cons as you list your priorities and do your research.

ADVANTAGES VERSUS DISADVANTAGES OF DAY CARE CENTERS

ADVANTAGES	DISADVANTAGES
They are often licensed or registered with the state.	Children are often exposed to illness from other babies.
Care is monitored by other staff and the day care director.	Noisy, busy environments can overstimulate babies.
Staff are often certified in CPR and first aid.	Having several providers can be confusing to your infant.
Staff often hold early childhood degrees or receive specialized training in child development.	Hours usually range from 6:00 A.M. to 6:00 P.M., without flexibility.
Educational programs are offered.	Staff turnover is high.
There are opportunities for babies to interact and socialize.	Formal day care centers are expensive.
When staff become ill, other providers can fill in.	

Before you make a decision about a formal day care center, ask the providers these questions:

- Is your center licensed or registered?
- What is the policy on the handling and storage of breastmilk?

- Is there a place I can nurse my baby after work or during breaks?
- What are your hours of operation?
- What is the cost?
- Are activities structured or child driven?
- How many children are cared for by each provider?
- Are staff trained in CPR and first aid?
- Is there clear communication between the center providers and parents in the form of conferences, flyers, or parent groups?
- What are your policies on discipline, emergencies, inclement weather, dispensing medications, and illness?
- Will I be charged if my infant is ill and absent from day care?

As you tour the center, pay special attention to the atmosphere and activities. Are rooms and toys clean and inviting? Are children engaged in developmentally appropriate activities? Do children seem happy? Are crying babies attended and soothed? Is the environment clean and safe for young children?

Don't be shy! Ask for references from other parents with infants the same age as your baby. Call them and ask them to describe the quality of care their babies receive in the center, as well as the pros and cons of placing children in this center's care. When you enroll, ask for copies of all policies and procedures, and get a copy of your contract. Day care is a business deal. Enter into it carefully.

Family Day Care Homes

Almost 40 percent of infants and toddlers in a day care setting are enrolled in family day care homes. Family day care is offered in the home of the primary provider, who usually has up to six children of varying ages in her care. Many new parents like the intimacy of family day care.

Many family day care homes are part of a network of child care resource and referral agencies. Some are part of human service organizations. Child care resource centers are listed in your phone book. They offer information about which day care homes in their network have openings, where they are located, what they charge, and whether they are registered or licensed.

ADVANTAGES VERSUS DISADVANTAGES OF FAMILY DAY CARE HOMES

ADVANTAGES	DISADVANTAGES
Child care occurs in a natural, home setting.	Alternative care may be unavailable if the provider is sick or on vacation.
Family day care homes are often inexpensive.	They are harder to monitor for quality of care.
Mixed-age groups allow children interactions through a variety of socialization experiences.	Some are not licensed or registered.
One consistent caregiver forms a relationship with your infant.	Children are exposed to illness.
Some providers offer flexible weekend and evening hours.	
Many are licensed or registered with the state.	

When considering the options of a family day care home, be just as clear in your expectations and priorities as you would at a "commercial" facility. Exercise your right to ask the provider these questions:

- Is your home licensed or registered?
- What is your policy on the handling and storage of breastmilk?
- Is space available to breastfeed my baby?
- How many children are in your care?
- Do you have backup support during family illness or vacation?
- Do you transport children in an insured vehicle? Do you have a valid driver's license?
- Are car seats available?
- Are you trained in CPR and first aid?
- What are your policies on discipline, emergencies, inclement weather, dispensing medications, and sick children?
- Can my baby still attend if he is ill?
- Is there still a charge if my infant is absent from day care?
- What are your hours of operation? Do you offer flexible hours?
- What is the cost?

Interview likely candidates more than once, and have your baby available for at least one of the interviews to observe his interaction with the provider and the provider's ease with your infant. You may also want to get a feel for your infant's ease with another care provider. Many infants may need time to get used to someone else, but at least you'll get a preview of what you can expect.

QUESTIONS?

When is the best time to visit a child care facility?
Schedule a tour of any day care home or center in the early morning or late afternoon. Most babies nap midmorning or after lunch. You want to observe activity and interaction between the provider and the children in her care.

Make a point to discuss parenting philosophies regarding such topics as breastfeeding, discipline, crying babies, colic, bonding, pacifier use, feeding styles, and potty learning with your intended provider. If the provider disagrees with your philosophies, find out whether she willing to accept and follow your preferences over her own.

In-Home Day Care

In-home care is an option that allows others to provide care for your baby in his own natural environment, his home. This kind of care can be expensive. Those with the financial resources often employ live-in nannies. A more cost-effective option for most would be to employ a friend or family member. Ask your friends, relatives, colleagues, neighbors, or acquaintances at your church to refer a skilled and dedicated in-home child care provider.

ESSENTIALS

If possible, arrange to be home with the provider for the first week, but keep a low profile. Your baby and the provider will need some time to get used to each other, while you'll get used to having a stranger care for your child.

ADVANTAGES VERSUS DISADVANTAGES OF IN-HOME CARE

ADVANTAGES	DISADVANTAGES
Your baby remains in familiar surroundings with all supplies needed for his care.	It's difficult to monitor the quality of care your infant receives.
Your baby receives consistency of care and full attention from one individual who will develop a relationship with him.	It's difficult to find someone outside of the family who can place the same investment in your child as you do.
Flexible hours may include evenings and weekends.	Alternative care if your in-home caregiver is sick may be difficult to find.
Your baby is not exposed to illness from other children.	It's a high-stress job and has high turnover rates (about 90 percent annually!).
Parents do not have to pack up little ones on cold mornings and transport them to day care.	It's expensive.
If a parent must travel, in-home care can provide around-the-clock supervision.	It can be isolating with little peer-group interaction for your growing baby.

Because you are dealing with an individual—a free agent, of sorts—you need to ask different questions and do additional and thorough research. Ask all candidates for an in-home care position these questions:

- What previous experience do you have with newborn care?
- What are the costs/fees involved?
- What special arrangements will you require (benefits, private room, evenings and weekends free)?
- Do you smoke, drink, or use drugs?
- Do you have transportation and a valid driver's license, and are you insured?
- Do you have any health concerns that might interfere with the job?
- Can you work flexible hours?
- Are there other children (her own) in your care?
- Can you provide full-time care, if needed?
- Why did you leave your last job?
- Have you ever been charged with a crime?

Ask for references and call them. Every one of them. Ask if they would hire this provider again. Were they pleased with the quality of care? Were there any concerns of which you should be aware?

Listen to your intuition when making a final decision. If something just doesn't seem right, you can either interview a third time or find another provider. You want to make the best decision based on all available information.

Breastfeeding and Day Care

Ask your provider not to feed your baby within an hour of when you plan to arrive. If your baby is hungry, ask your provider to feed her just enough to take the edge off of her appetite. That means you'll need to have extra breastmilk available at the day care, especially if your baby receives human milk exclusively. Formula supplements take longer to digest and your baby might not be hungry when you arrive to nurse her.

SSENTIALS

If you've established a sound breastfeeding routine and you think your baby is ready for a pacifier, you can ask your provider to offer your baby her "plug" throughout the day. This will help meet her need to suck and might stave off hunger until you arrive.

Many babies suffer from nipple confusion when they are not used to supplements or expressed milk in a bottle. The milk smells like their mother's, but the containers and nipples are different. Some babies adamantly refuse the bottle. They will let go of the nipple, thrash their heads, reattach, get frustrated, and cry.

Practice using a bottle for a few feedings before the first day of day care. Babies can also be cup fed, spoon fed, or offered milk in a feeding syringe. Older infants can use a straw or sippy cup. Work closely with your provider to develop a feeding system that works for everyone.

Other causes for feeding difficulties at day care include a change of environment, noise levels, different smells, and constant activity. Talk to your child care provider about your baby's feeding schedules. Remember that your baby will eat when he's hungry and will stop when he's full.

Returning to Work

Almost half of the U.S. work force is female. Because of this, special considerations are now being given to make breastfeeding and employment more compatible.

Returning to work should be a gradual process. Talk to your employer before you start maternity leave. Discuss the possibility of returning at part-time status or for half-days for the first few weeks back. Ask if you can return on a Thursday or Friday, creating a long transitional weekend to get mentally prepared and back on track. Other options to consider include job sharing, working from home, or flexible scheduling. Some small businesses might allow your young, nonmobile infant to come to work with you. Research the policies or benefits that are offered for breastfeeding women.

Breastfeeding-Friendly Employment Environments

Being family-friendly is good business and good for business! What makes a company family-friendly? Consider companies that:

- Offer paid parental leave or give options to take longer unpaid parental leaves without the threat of job loss
- Offer on-site child care or partner with community child care providers
- Provide nursing breaks for breastfeeding moms (two thirty-minute breaks, plus lunch) and provide lactation rooms where mothers can express and store their milk
- Provide subsidies for breast pump rental, or offer lactation consultation through community collaboration

While this may sound expensive to an employer, it's really to the company's advantage. Offering these kinds of benefits decreases employee absenteeism and turnover. Maintaining qualified personnel by offering lactation rooms returns a huge payoff. Babies who are breastfed get sick less often, so parents use fewer sick days. Employees feel supported and valued. They have higher morale and productivity, enhanced loyalty to their company, and lower insurance claims. It also improves the company's position and respectability in the community.

Maintaining Your Milk Supply

Begin to stockpile your milk for at least a week before returning to work. Express on the weekends and throughout the day, just as you would after your baby nurses.

As you pump milk at work, you might notice a decrease in production during the first week. This is normal. You'll continue to produce an abundant supply if you follow a regular pumping schedule and nurse your baby frequently when you return home. She can empty the breast more efficiently that any breast pump can.

FACTS

You may encounter colleagues who seem resentful of the time you are spending expressing your milk, especially if they have to assume your responsibilities while you are away from your desk. Don't take this to heart. Show your appreciation to coworkers by sending them a thank-you note signed by your baby.

Nurse early in the morning, then again before you leave for work. Your milk supply is most abundant in the mornings when you have higher levels of prolactin. Express milk throughout the day, and nurse your baby again when you pick him up from day care. Many child care providers offer a quiet space to nurse your baby. They can also have your baby awake and ready to nurse when you arrive if you call in advance.

Staying Home

Research findings conclude that returning to work is correlated with decreased breastfeeding rates, but making the decision not to return to work can be difficult. Most women believe they must work for financial reasons. However, many have found that staying home with their child is less of a financial sacrifice than they feared. The often-overlooked truth of the matter is that most families' second incomes are far less profitable than they think. We see the figure on our paychecks but don't always fully consider how much is spent in related costs.

One study by the U.S. Department of Labor found that about 80 percent of a working mother's income is absorbed by job-related expenses. So, if you earn $25,000 annually, your actual take-home pay might be around $5,000. That's just over $400 per month. It's not even unusual for couples to discover that their second income is entirely consumed by work-related expenses.

Here are a few factors to consider in making a decision about returning to work or staying home.

Career paths. Many women have invested a great deal of time and effort into their careers and enjoy working too much to consider staying home. You might decide that your career goals would be compromised by an interruption. Your needs and desires are always an important consideration.

Clothing and transportation expenses. The cost of commuting can be substantial whether you drive, take the bus, or carpool. For some urban families, one vehicle would be enough if not for the second job. Car payments, tolls, parking, gas, and service all add up. Then there's the cost of maintaining a professional wardrobe. You'll still need dressy clothes for some occasions, but not as many and they'll last longer.

Cost of day care. Day care can be expensive. You can expect to pay at least $700 to $1,000 per month for infant care, depending on what type you choose. As discussed earlier, family day care homes are the least expensive, and in-home care is the most expensive. If you have more than one child, expenses could double.

Food expenses at work versus home. Unless you're the kind of person who packs an inexpensive sack lunch every day, workday food expenses can really put a dent in your pocketbook. The average homemade lunch costs less than $1. The cheapest fast-food meal is more than twice that. That's over $250 per year, not counting trips to the vending machine for snacks. The other, often hidden, food expense to consider is the cost of ordering out at night because everyone is too tired or impatient to prepare a meal.

Health insurance. You need to have health insurance. Babies get sick from time to time and health insurance is a wonderful benefit most employers offer. Well-child visits during the first three years of life will outnumber those needed for the ten years following. A trip to the doctor's office can easily set you back $150 or more, depending on what treatment is medically indicated. Most insurance companies offer copays for as little as $10 per visit.

Intellectual stimulation and camaraderie. Staying at home can be very isolating and even boring at times. Your baby is always happy to interact with you, but sometimes you'll miss adult conversation and the friendly camaraderie of your fellow employees. Many stay-at-home parents start playgroups, write newsletters, take up hobbies, and volunteer at schools to combat feelings of isolation.

Self-esteem and social status. Many people define themselves in terms of what they do. Losing that role can leave some parents feeling depressed or diminished. There's a real lack of appreciation in the world for the hard work, skill, and ingenuity of stay-at-home parents.

Taxes from a second income. All the taxes deducted from your paycheck need to be taken into account to discover its true take-home value. If your second income puts the family into a higher tax bracket than your primary income alone would, then you have to figure the extra taxes paid on the primary income as expenses related to the secondary income. In plain English, if the second income puts the family into a 22 percent tax bracket when it would otherwise be in an 18 percent bracket, the extra 4 percent taken out of one check is an expense related to the second.

Time. Time is money, so they say. Much of the expense of the dual-income lifestyle originates in lost time. You don't have time to paint the living room, so you hire a painter. You don't have time to cook, so you order out. You don't have time to shop for the best prices, so you buy whatever you can get quickly. Convenience is the hot new benefit offered in today's marketplace, and it costs money. Moderately careful stay-at-home parents can sometimes save more than they would earn at a regular job, simply by investing their time wisely.

Ifyou find that your job is less profitable than you thought, maybe it's time to consider becoming a full-time parent for a while. On the other hand, if you're unableto stay home, there are other solutions. You could job share, work part-time, or conduct business out of a home office.

JOB-RELATED EXPENSES WORKSHEET	
Taxes (Taken from your check and possibly your partner's)	$_____
Work Clothing (Purchase price, wear, dry cleaning)	$_____
Transportation (Car payment, parking, fuel, insurance)	$_____
Eating Out/Snacks (List only the difference over home cooking.)	$_____
Day care	$_____
Office Gifts (Birthdays, funeral flowers, etc.)	$_____
Convenience Services (Things you could do if you had time)	$_____
Total Expenses:	$_____
Gross Income:	$_____
Value of Your Job (Income – expenses):	$_____

Stay-at-Home Dads

More and more fathers are moving away from employment outside the home to full-time fathering and housekeeping. An estimated 2 million fathers stay at home and care for their children while Mom goes off to work. It's an arrangement that benefits the entire family. Mothers can continue on their career paths uninterrupted, knowing that their children are being cared for by someone who loves them. Fathers can enjoy the special parent-child relationship that usually belongs to Mom.

FACTS

Sixty-five percent of stay-at-home fathers surveyed, and 78 percent of their spouses, chose their arrangement because they wanted their child to be raised by a parent. The secondary reason in many of the studied cases was financial. The mothers made more money, a situation that's no longer unusual in the United States.

Rather than having a simple reversal of household roles, families with stay-at-home dads tend to be more balanced. Parental power and responsibilities are more evenly divided than in more traditional family arrangements.

Couples considering this move need to consider all the factors listed earlier, paying special attention to the social and emotional criteria. There aren't very many traditional role models for stay-at-home fathers. Studies show that the isolation of staying home and the loss of self-esteem and status from leaving their jobs hits men harder than it hits women.

However, staying home with your child is a richly rewarding experience that few people of either gender would fail to appreciate. Fortunately for men, it's an opportunity that's becoming more common every day.

CHAPTER 22

Breastfeeding and the Law

More and more lawmakers realize the importance of breastfeeding. State, local, and federal officials are leading the way with new laws that are designed to provide support and encouragement for breastfeeding mothers. They know that breastfeeding is vital to the health and well-being of families everywhere. You have a well-established right to breastfeed your baby for as long as you want and, generally, wherever you want.

Nursing in Public

In the United States, breastfeeding is your right. However, on occasion someone will ask a woman not to nurse her baby in some particular setting. You should know that the courts have put no such restrictions on breastfeeding. Breastfeeding is not indecent exposure. It is a natural and healthy way for a mother to feed her child.

As a rule, you're permitted to nurse your child anywhere you have a legal right to be. That means at the library, the mall, a restaurant, or anywhere else that the public in general, or you in particular, is free to visit. Further, you're not restricted to the use of a special area while nursing. They can't shuffle you off to a bathroom or a table in the back if you don't want to go.

That right was highlighted by the U.S. Congress in 1999. The Treasury and General Government Appropriations Act was signed into law by President Clinton. Part of that Act protected women's right to breastfeed their children on any federally owned property.

Twenty-eight states have also passed legislation that clarifies a woman's right to breastfeed anywhere in public. Those states are:

Alaska	Illinois	Montana	Oregon
California	Iowa	Nevada	Rhode Island
Connecticut	Louisiana	New Hampshire	Texas
Delaware	Maine	New Jersey	Utah
Florida	Michigan	New Mexico	Virginia
Georgia	Minnesota	New York	Washington
Hawaii	Missouri	North Carolina	Wisconsin

Three states place restrictions on a mother's right to breastfeed. The most common restriction is one calling for discretion. While many states specifically allow the breast or nipple to be visible during breastfeeding, two states are less liberal. Most women are unlikely to have a problem with a request for modesty, but including such restrictions in the law could have a chilling effect on breastfeeding in general.

California law reiterates your right to nurse your child in any place you have the right to be with one exception. For some reason, the legislators found it necessary to specifically exclude any private home that a breastfeeding mother might be visiting.

Georgia supports a woman's right to nurse her baby in public but requires that she be discreet and modest. Those restrictions are currently coming under attack in the state legislature. There is the possibility that the legislature will remove the requirements for discretion by amendment.

Missouri requires that breastfeeding moms use as much discretion as possible when nursing in public, but otherwise sets no restrictions.

At the other end of the spectrum, three states actually go so far as to specify punishment for those who attempt to limit public nursing.

Connecticut mandates a fine of $25 to $100 for anyone interfering with a breastfeeding mother's right to nurse her child in public. The courts also have the option of imprisoning the offender for up to thirty days in jail.

Hawaii provides penalties for anyone discriminating against a nursing mother. A $100 fine plus court costs may be levied. In addition, the offended mother is authorized to pursue her case in court.

New Jersey sets forth a fine of $25 to $200 for anyone interfering with a mother's right to breastfeed her child in public.

Two states pioneered the way in public breastfeeding.

Florida started the current trend of breastfeeding legislation in 1993. Florida's law was the first to specifically exclude public breastfeeding from any criminal prosecution (for indecent exposure).

New York was the first state to include breastfeeding of children as a civil right. In some situations, mothers serving a prison sentence are permitted to nurse their children below one year of age.

If you are asked to stop nursing your child in public, you might be embarrassed at first. Stay confident, knowing that you are nurturing your child in the best possible way and that the law is on your side. If you live in a state that has passed public nursing legislation, inform your critic of the law.

The Workplace

There are probably few things as generally unpleasant as sitting in a toilet stall at work over your lunch break, pumping milk for your baby. That's dedication! Fortunately, things are changing for breastfeeding moms on the job all over the country. Employers are being educated on how maintaining a breastfeeding-friendly workplace benefits everyone.

The following states require employers to support their breastfeeding employees:

Connecticut provides that women be allowed to breastfeed or express milk during meal or break times. Employers are prohibited from discriminating against breastfeeding employees. Employers also have to make a reasonable effort to provide a private place near the work site for breastfeeding activities except in cases where that would create "undue hardship" for the employer.

Minnesota was the first state to make employers accommodate breastfeeding mothers who were returning to work.

Tennessee was the second state to require that breastfeeding employees be accommodated in the workplace.

Hawaii bans discrimination of lactating women in the workplace. Employers are required to allow moms to breastfeed or pump during their regular breaks and mealtimes.

Illinois requires employers to accommodate the needs of their breastfeeding employees.

California passed a law in October 2001 requiring employers to provide adequate time and facilities for employees who are breastfeeding or expressing milk.

New York is currently considering a bill to protect lactation in the workplace.

Four other states have addressed the issue in less direct ways.

California has a resolution that encourages all employers to support breastfeeding by providing adequate facilities for nursing or pumping.

Florida has legislation that encourages employers to support breastfeeding.

Texas law allows employers to advertise themselves as "breastfeeding-friendly" if they meet certain criteria.

Washington encourages employers to support breastfeeding by allowing them to call themselves "infant-friendly" if they meet certain criteria.

Congress is currently considering several bills that would affect how breastfeeding is supported in the workplace. New York Representative Carolyn Maloney has introduced bills that would protect lactating women from discrimination under federal civil rights laws as well as encourage and reward employer accommodation of lactating employees. Another current bill is the Federal Employees Paid Parental Leave Act. That Act would grant six weeks of paid leave to a new parent. If passed, these new federal laws will have an incredibly positive impact on the health and happiness of American working families.

Family Law

Divorce or separation can wreak havoc on your breastfeeding relationship. As if the inevitable stress isn't destructive enough, mother and child might be faced with a court-ordered custody or visitation schedule that makes regular breastfeeding next to impossible. Most courts are reluctant to reduce a father's time with his child for the sake of breastfeeding, believing that both parents have an important part to play in a child's life. Only three states currently require that breastfeeding issues be considered in family-law situations.

Maine requires courts to consider breastfeeding issues when deciding on matters of separation or divorce involving children under one year of age.

Michigan requires judges to consider breastfeeding when ruling on family-law cases.

Utah courts consider breastfeeding when setting up custody and visitation rights for parents, especially when those cases involve children less than eighteen months of age.

ESSENTIALS   If you find yourself separated from your child for many hours, or even a day or two, you can still continue to breastfeed. You'll have to pump in addition to nursing your baby in order to build up a surplus of frozen breastmilk you can send along on your baby's visits with his father.

Although most states don't expressly require that breastfeeding be considered, judges generally want to know of any circumstances affecting your child's health and emotional well-being. Try to keep your comments positive and recognize the court's interest in keeping your partner involved, no matter what you might be feeling about him right now.

Family and Medical Leave Act (FMLA)

The Family and Medical Leave Act (FMLA) has been a blessing to countless thousands of American families. Thanks to the FMLA, many working men and women in the United States are able to take time off from their jobs for pregnancy and newborn care without fear of losing their jobs or even their health insurance. The U.S. Congress passed the Act in 1992 and it went into effect nationwide in 1993–1994.

The FMLA allows eligible employees to take up to twelve weeks of unpaid leave from their jobs for certain specific family or medical reasons within a twelve-month period. The twelve-month period can be the calendar year, an employer-specified fixed leave or fiscal year, or the twelve months before or after the beginning of your leave.

Qualification

To find out if you qualify for Family Leave under the Act, let's play Survivor: The FMLA Edition. You get to bring just one thing from home to help you in the game. We suggest it be your family.

The object of the game is to be left standing after meeting all of the challenges. Unlike the real Survivor, you won't be alone. About 50 percent of American workers are covered by the FMLA.

Challenge One

You won't be eating any disgusting "foods" or playing any weird mind games with the other contestants, but there might be times when those things don't sound so hard in comparison. Okay, here we go.

If you . . .

- Are giving birth or caring for your newborn child
- Are adopting a child or accepting a child for foster care
- Care for a spouse, child, or parent with a serious health condition
- Need time off because of your own serious health condition

. . . then you've made it past the first FMLA Survivor challenge. Get ready for your next challenge.

Challenge Two

They've had Survivor in Australia, Africa, and on an island in the Pacific, but FMLA Survivor is played in the workplace. In one version, you face snakes, exhaustion, and dirty tricks surrounded by strangers. In the other, you're thousands of miles from home in an exotic locale. This next challenge is designed to weed out the individuals who don't qualify for an FMLA leave because of their employer.

If you . . .

- Work for a public agency, including local schools or state, local, and federal government
- Work for a private employer who has at least fifty employees during at least twenty or more work weeks in the current or preceding calendar year

. . . then you've made it through another harrowing tribal council. You're going on to the final level.

But, if you're employed by a small, independently owned business, the FMLA probably doesn't apply to you. Likewise, if you work for a new start-up business that's been around for only a few months, you might have to wait a while before you can take your leave.

You've been a wonderful contestant, but the tribe has spoken. Please extinguish your ceremonial torch on your way out.

Challenge Three

Now things get a little more personal. This challenge examines the nature of your job.

If you . . .

- Have worked for your employer for a total of twelve months, and
- Have worked at least 1,250 hours in those twelve months (full-time employment is 2,000 hours annually, figured at forty hours per week, 50 weeks per year), and
- Work in the United States or in a territory or possession of the United States where at least fifty employees are employed by your employer within seventy-five miles

. . . then congratulations! You've won! You don't get a million dollars, but you do get twelve weeks of quality time with your baby. If you didn't make it past this round, take heart. You're not alone. Almost half of the work force didn't make it, just like you.

And now for the fine print:

- Leave taken for newborn care or adoptive or foster care must end within twelve months from the date of birth, adoption, or placement.
- Spouses who work for the same employer will receive a combined total of twelve weeks' leave, not twelve weeks each.
- Unless medically necessary, FMLA leave is ordinarily taken in a single block of time. If your employer approves, leave can be taken intermittently or by reducing the number of hours in your workweek.

FACTS

The FMLA defines "serious health condition" as an illness, injury, impairment, or condition that involves a hospital stay or any of the following:

1. A condition that lasts at least three consecutive days or requires treatment aimed at preventing an incapacity of more than three days
2. Pregnancy
3. A long-term, serious condition requiring visits to a health care provider that might involve occasional incapacity
4. A permanent or long-term condition that might not respond to treatment

If you have any questions about your company's policies and philosophies, talk to your manager and your company's human resource department. Know your rights, and maintain open lines of communication with your employer to ensure a positive experience for all parties.

Planning Your Leave

Whenever possible, you are required to give your employer thirty days' notice of your intent to take FMLA leave. It's usually a good idea to give notice as far in advance as possible, even beyond thirty days. Your boss will appreciate the extra time to make alternate arrangements.

Your employer is required to let you know what you have to do with regard to your leave. You may be asked to provide medical certification of your reason for leave, second or third medical opinions (at your company's expense), and even periodic reports throughout the leave. Those reports can include information on your health and your desire to return to work.

ALERT

There are at least two circumstances when the FMLA itself requires that you consider how your leave impacts your employer. One is for planned medical treatment that could be scheduled anytime. The other is for employees of local schools.

It's in everyone's best interest to work together to ensure that your leave works for you and your family, but always make a reasonable effort to take your employer's needs into consideration. It will help smooth the way for your friendly return and keeps the doors open for others in your workplace to enjoy the same benefit.

Financial Considerations

The loss of pay during your leave under the Act can be a real problem. You should know that federal guidelines allow either employers or employees to use accrued paid leave time to cover a portion of the FMLA absence (up to the entire length of the leave). If you choose to use your paid leave time as compensation for your FMLA leave, you'll need to work out the details with your employer.

Your health insurance is protected under the FMLA, but you're still responsible for any portion of the expense of that insurance you would normally pay.

You should also know that if you decide to quit your job after your leave, your employer can demand reimbursement for any portion of your health insurance premiums that the organization paid during your FMLA absence.

Back to Work

When you return to work from your leave, your employer is usually required to give you either your last position, or an equivalent position with no loss of status or benefits. However, where the employer can show that giving you your job back would cause serious economic harm to the operation, it might not have to follow through. If you are a salaried individual among the top 10 percent of employees within seventy-five miles of your work site, the organization might not have to take you back. So you won't be caught off guard in that situation, the Act requires that employers:

1. Notify you of your status as a "key" employee when you tell them you plan to take FMLA leave;
2. Notify you as soon as they decide they will deny your job restoration, and explain the reasons for the decision;

3. Offer you a reasonable time to return to work after telling you they don't plan to take you back;

4. Withhold final determination until the end of your leave, if you ask to be reinstated.

The FMLA is not optional for most employers. If the company you work for or any of its representatives interferes with, restrains, or denies the exercise of any right provided by FMLA, they are in violation of federal law. They can't fire or discriminate against any employee who opposes any practice or takes part in any process related to the FMLA.

Lobbying for Change

When Americans feel they've been wronged, they go to court. However, civil cases alleging discrimination based on breastfeeding haven't been very successful in the past.

If you feel your rights under the FMLA have been denied, contact the Wage and Hour Division of the U.S. Department of Labor. You also have the right to bring a private civil action against an employer for violations.

Instead, try to educate the people around you on breastfeeding issues. Most people simply don't realize the importance of breastfeeding. Don't preach, just chat about it in a positive, friendly way.

If you'd like to see new breastfeeding-friendly laws on the books, whether nationally or locally, you can do it! Contact your council member, representative, congressional representative, or senator. Make your voice heard.

If Washington, D.C., seems too far away and too slow, start locally. You can make a difference!

CHAPTER 23
Weaning

When to wean depends on both you and your baby. Some babies lose interest in nursing once solids are offered or the cup is introduced. Others nurse happily until they become mobile and begin to move toward independence. Still others are content to nurse throughout their preschool years. The methods you use will differ depending on who's initiating the process.

Nursing Strike versus Weaning

Sometimes, completely out of the blue, a baby decides he doesn't want to nurse. He'll purse his lips, refuse the breast, and cry. This might last for one feeding or for several days. It can be hard to tell if your baby is ill, self-weaning, or holding a nursing strike.

Many moms mistake a nursing strike for self-weaning and give up breastfeeding long before their babies are ready. Babies who self-wean usually lose interest gradually over time or are more distractible at the breast. In contrast, most nursing strikes happen suddenly and while babies are still very young.

QUESTIONS?

What might cause a nursing strike?
Babies choose not to nurse for a variety of reasons. Teething can be a big factor. Also, swallowing and jaw movement might be painful for your baby if he's suffering from an earache, mouth injury, or sore throat. Maybe your baby senses stress or anxiety. Even changes like a new deodorant or perfume can cause confusion.

The solution? If at first you don't succeed, try, try again. Offer the breast when your baby is sleepy. He is less prone to fight it when he's tired. Offer to nurse again as your baby wakes. The quiet-alert state is best. Some suggest that simply changing feeding positions or nursing while walking helps.

If your baby still refuses to nurse, express your milk and offer it in an infant feeding cup, a spoon, a syringe, an eyedropper, or a sippy cup.

Your milk supply is regulated by your baby's demand. When your baby refuses to nurse, your body slows production. Nursing strikes usually don't exceed beyond four days, but by that time, your milk supply could decrease. To maintain your supply, express milk manually or with a breast pump as often as your baby would normally nurse.

After twenty-four hours of baby's refusal of the breast, it's time to call your doctor or lactation consultant. Your baby might need a checkup to factor out health conditions like thrush or ear infection.

SSENTIALS

Remember: Your baby is not rejecting you; he is temporarily rejecting the breast. In a short while, the cause of the strike will resolve and you'll resume your breastfeeding relationship.

Special Situations: Sudden Weaning

Abrupt weaning can be difficult and uncomfortable for both mother and baby. It can lead to engorgement and breast infections, as well as feelings of depression and loss for Mom. It can also lead to nipple confusion if your baby is transitioned to a bottle for the first time.

Teething and the Breast

Teething can hurt—especially when teeth are coming in like popcorn. The process can disrupt the breastfeeding relationship if it's simply too painful for your baby to nurse. Your baby might refuse the breast or she might bite you to help work her teeth through. The initial shock and pain might cause you to reflexively shout, which will, in turn, scare your baby and might cause her to refuse the breast the next time it's offered.

ALERT

Sudden weaning can cause clogged ducts or breast infection. See your doctor or midwife if you experience fever, chills, heat in your breast, or flulike symptoms. You may need to be treated with an antibiotic.

If you're aware of the signs of teething, you can be on guard against biting before it happens. Signs of teething include:

- Biting everything in sight from spoons and sippy cup lids to you and unsuspecting playmates
- Diaper rash from diahrrea caused by the acids in excess saliva
- Drooling
- Rash or chapped chin
- Tearfulness

Teething does not have to be a reason to wean, although many parents use this event as a time to transition babies to the bottle.

The Emotional Rollercoaster

As prolactin levels decrease, you may begin to experience a temporary bout of baby blues. Baby blues are characterized by feelings of sadness, teariness, decrease in appetite, confusion, insomnia, and mood swings. You might have put off this postpartum phenomenon because you made the decision to breastfeed. But with sudden weaning you may begin to experience these symptoms for the first time.

These feelings will pass as your hormones balance out, but it's important to eat right, exercise, take time for yourself, and find a supportive person to talk to.

Stopping Your Milk Production

Stopping breastfeeding cold turkey is usually an unnecessary process. Ideally, weaning is a gradual process. When you wean suddenly, the results can be painful.

Engorgement caused by rapid weaning can leave you with full, painful breasts. When this happens, express just enough milk to make yourself comfortable, but remember that milk is made by supply and demand. When you express milk, it will be replaced with more. Milk remaining in the breast signals your body that you have more milk than you're using, and will slow production.

There are several other methods you can use to decrease milk production and the pain of engorgement.

Cabbage Leaves

Earlier, you learned that cool cabbage leaves tucked into your bra can relieve engorgment. You also learned not to use them too long or too often because they slow milk production. Now your goal is to slow production, so feel free to use them as much as you need to.

Leaves should be changed when they begin to wilt. During weaning, cabbage leaves can be worn around the clock.

Estrogen

Estrogen, as discussed earlier, is a hormone that reduces milk production. Some birth control pills contain high levels of estrogen, which will decrease your milk supply. However, many birth control pills on the market today are estrogen-free. Talk to your doctor before asking for a prescription. Estrogen has been associated with breast cancer, as well as uterine and cervical cancers, so making a decision to take these for weaning may be difficult.

Herbs and Medications

In our own mothers' day, medications were prescribed to reduce milk supply and engorgement. Many doctors no longer recommend medications because of the risk of serious side effects. Parlodel, for example, is no longer approved by the FDA, because it can cause seizures, strokes, and heart attacks. Ask your doctor about the side effects of every medication she recommends.

Sage tea has been used to help reduce milk supply. But herbs, like medications, also have side effects. Don't begin new herbal therapies while your baby is still nursing. Chemical compounds in the herbs find their way into your breastmilk, and from there, into your baby. Talk to your doctor, midwife, or lactation consultant first.

Transitioning Baby: Gradual Weaning

Gradual weaning begins with a plan. Look at a calendar to put this in perspective. You'll need six to eight weeks for a comfortable transition. The more time you take, the less traumatic it will be for both you and your child.

Gradual weaning will help you maintain a healthy hormonal balance. Because your hormone levels will decrease more slowly over time, you'll feel fewer symptoms of the baby blues. The key to keeping mood swings in check is proceeding slowly.

A gradual transition will also keep lactation in balance. Mothers who wean slowly don't experience engorgement. Your weaning infant or toddler will help your body produce just the right amount of milk.

Reduced Feedings

When is your baby least interested in nursing? Midmorning? Early evening? Those will be the first feedings to eliminate, but only one at a time. If you decide to wean in two months, plot out sessions to eliminate, as well as new activities or foods to substitute.

Keep an eye on toddlers who are slow to accept change. Weaning can be scary and stressful for them. Avoid emotional battles over the breast. Slow-to-transition children need more time to accept change. Flexibility is important!

Decrease your nursing schedule by one session every five days. For example, eliminate midmorning nursing, and after five days, begin to eliminate early evening sessions. Bedtimes and naptimes will be the last to go because babies often suck for comfort on these occasions. Nighttime feedings are usually the most difficult to give up. Patience and consistency are key. Inconsistency will only delay the process.

Offer the breast less frequently and for shorter amounts of time. A delayed nursing session might even make a busy toddler forget. Don't refuse your child the breast, but don't offer it frequently.

Change Routines

When it's time to eliminate that final nursing session of the day, rethink the bedtime routine. Give your baby a bath, read a story, drink a cup of water, brush her teeth, put on a lullaby tape, give a brief massage, kiss, and say goodnight. If you've weaned to the bottle, let Dad offer a bottle of water and initiate the bedtime routine.

Your partner can also spend time alone with your weaning baby. An afternoon out together, a walk around the block, or cuddling during storytime will distract a busy toddler from wanting the breast.

It's often helpful to eliminate the feeding-cues that remind your baby that it's time to nurse. Sit on the couch instead of the chair. Face baby forward in the sling rather than toward your breast.

If your baby is six months of age, offer her a sippy cup with expressed breastmilk, 100 percent fruit juice, or water. A new taste, along with the novelty of the cup, will appeal to her. You can also replace a nursing session with the introduction of a new solid food. But remember to try new foods one at a time, and watch for signs of allergy.

Offer the cup following a feeding of solids and expect a mess. Remember: Babies are moist and they learn through their senses. Wet is good to a baby. Slidey, squishy, squirmy wet is even better.

QUESTIONS?

What's the best way to get your baby used to a cup?
Begin to introduce the cup between six and nine months of age. Babies develop the ability to move objects from hand to hand in the middle of their bodies (midline) at around six months. By nine months, this skill is well mastered and babies are ready to manipulate cups with lids.

Expect the cup to become a new toy for your baby. He'll throw it and expect you to pick it up (over and over and over). This game is not played to frustrate you, nor is it a sign of sippy cup palsy. Your baby is learning cause and effect ("If I throw it, you'll pick it up . . . every time!") and object permanence (out of sight is not out of mind). Both of these concepts are important for normal development, and you've just provided the right age-appropriate toy to teach them.

Gradual Weaning by Age

Your weaning plan should take into account your child's age and developmental abilities. A child who is moving toward independence is more distractible than a child who has a much more predictable routine.

Think about the ages and stages of your child when developing your weaning plan.

0 to 6 months: Wean from the breast to a bottle. Babies still have a need to suck. To avoid battles, offer the bottle to your baby when he is neither too tired nor too hungry. Babies at this age will often experience nipple confusion. Vary feeding positions, try different bottle nipples, and have someone else offer the bottle if he rejects it from you.

6 to 12 months: You can gradually replace breastfeeding sessions with solid foods and the introduction of the cup. Offer the cup more frequently. A pacifier can meet your baby's need to suck. Infants at this age are more distractible. A change in routines can help them transition from the breast more easily.

12 to 24 months: Your toddler is moving toward independence and is mastering self-help skills. Toddlers at this age can now successfully manipulate a cup. Use the cup more frequently and begin to offer water in the bottle, if your child is using one. Your toddler is now eating table foods and has a varied diet. He sleeps through the night and doesn't rely on late-night feedings. This is the ideal age to introduce transitional objects for security (teddy bears and blankets) and to wean from the bottle. Teach your baby other ways to comfort himself.

24 to 36 months: Toddlers are active, curious, and on the go! You can substitute activities, like trips to the zoo or playground, in place of nursing. A change in routine will help eliminate nursing cues. Use a cup during cuddle times. Children love to listen to stories and make up their own. Replace nursing sessions with lap time in a different chair.

36 months and over: Children at this age nurse for emotional closeness. They prefer to play but still need to feel the safety of their parents. Invite friends over to play more frequently. Have Dad offer days out with your preschooler as a change in routine.

If you have concerns with your baby's development with respect to his age, discuss your weaning options or plan with your pediatrician or lactation consultant. Again, you know your child best and are the most qualified judge of what methods will work for you and your family.

Weaning from Breast to Bottle

Introduction to the bottle should be a gradual process. Bottle nipples aren't like human nipples, and infants suck differently from breast to bottle to cup. The nipple flow from a bottle releases milk more quickly, and depending on the nipple, in larger quantities. Look for signs of gulping and sputtering when your infant swallows. This indicates that the nipple flow is too fast. Switch to a slow-flow nipple (like NUK or Avent) or replace your current bottle nipple with a newborn size and flow rate.

Bottle-fed babies are more prone to ear infections. As you begin to wean from breast to bottle, feed formula or expressed milk midevening and water before bedtime. Milk that collects in the eustachian tubes is a perfect host for bacteria that will lead to painful ear infections.

Many babies experience nipple confusion when transitioning from breast to bottle. Often they'll refuse to take a bottle from their mother. Although the milk tastes and smells the same, the containers are different.

Transitioning off the breast is a perfect opportunity for Dad to begin feeding his baby. Ask him to offer milk or formula in a bottle or a cup.

Weaning from the Bottle

Weaning from the bottle usually happens somewhere between nine months and two years of age. Older infants and toddlers are often reluctant to give up the bottle because it soothes them to sleep and provides a "safety zone" for times of anxiety in a big and busy world.

Some parents use the water technique to wean from the bottle. Water is substituted for milk at bedtimes and naptimes, when busy babies and young toddlers seem to want the bottle most often. Because water is less attractive, babies give it up more quickly. If you plan to use this technique, expect some initial resistance. As with all parenting decisions, choose your battles wisely and be consistent once a rule is established.

SSENTIALS Keep some perspective on the use of the bottle as a method of feeding your infant. Make yourself, and not the bottle, available to him for physical and emotional comfort throughout the day.

Natural Weaning

Natural weaning is a child-driven process. It happens in baby steps usually between the ages of twelve months and three years. When you allow your toddler to set the rhythm, weaning happens naturally. Your hormone levels decline more slowly. There is little risk of baby blues or breast engorgement.

A child's readiness to wean brings closure to the breastfeeding experience. When he initiates the process at his own pace, there are fewer power struggles. It allows him to have a greater sense of control and nurtures his self-esteem.

FACTS Did you know that some mothers can still express breastmilk long after they've weaned their babies or toddlers? In fact, some mothers still have small amounts of milk for up to two or more years following the weaning of their baby! It is not unusual and not cause for alarm.

Mobile infants and toddlers are easily distracted by outside stimuli and will often wean themselves as they become more independent. While it's important to encourage your child's independence, it's equally important to meet his emotional needs. This is the "Don't offer, don't refuse" stage of weaning. If your toddler requests to nurse, you can allow it as often and for as long as you wish. But if you don't offer, your busy toddler will find other diversions.

Other Bonding Activities

As they transition from the breast, babies still need to be close to their loving parents, both physically and emotionally. Let your baby know you're available to him in other ways besides breastfeeding. He needs the comfort of his mother's arms and plenty of time to cuddle.

Here are a few activities that will continue your nurturing relationship. (In fact, you may find that these activities are good for all nurturing relationships!)

- Color or draw together
- Cuddle
- Dance
- Do fingerplays
- Go on a field trip
- Laugh at funny faces
- Listen to music
- Offer massage
- Read or tell stories to each other
- Recite nursery rhymes
- Rock in a chair
- Sing songs
- Tickle each other

Breastfeeding gave your child the most natural and healthy start to his or her life, but that was only the beginning. You'll spend the rest of your lives concerned with the health and welfare of your children as they continue to grow, learn, and become more independent every day. Through all the challenges that come with raising a family, have faith in yourself and your abilities, and remember, above all, to be loving and patient.

Frequently Asked Questions

The information provided in the following pages is addressed in greater detail within the body of *The Everything® Breastfeeding Book*. FAQs will provide an excellent review of breastfeeding in general, and may highlight some of your specific concerns. If you or your baby has specialized needs, speak with your OB, pediatrician, or lactation consultant. These professionals can offer you the best advice, based on your personal situation.

Q: My breasts are small. Can I still breastfeed?

A: Breast size is not an indicator of your ability to produce milk. However, if you've had breast reduction surgery or have undeveloped breast tissue, talk to your doctor.

Q: Will it hurt?

A: Breastfeeding will help relieve the pain of engorgement, which will happen whether you breastfeed or not. There may be some very mild discomfort during the first week while your baby is learning to latch on properly, but it is temporary and not painful.

Q: My family wants a chance to feed the baby from a bottle. What should I do?

A: It's important that your baby breastfeed exclusively for the first six weeks to ensure strong milk production and to avoid nipple confusion. Encourage your family to bond with your baby in other ways, like bathing, snuggling, rocking, and infant massage.

Q: Can I breastfeed if my nipples are pierced and/or I have breast tattoos?

A: Most women with pierced nipples can breastfeed without problems, but you should remove your jewelry first. Pierced nipples also tend to leak. Tattoo dyes do not penetrate into the milk-producing cells.

Q: Why should I breastfeed?

A: Human milk has been perfected over millions of years of evolution for babies. It is a vital part of a baby's immunity against disease and is easier to digest than other animal milk or artificial formula. Also, breastfeeding provides a woman with some degree of protection against breast cancer. Breastfeeding is a nutritious, emotionally satisfying, and economical practice.

Q: Will breastfeeding make my breasts sag?

A: No, heredity, pregnancy, and age cause breasts to sag.

Q: How can I breastfeed and go back to work?

A: Many women continue nursing their babies after they return to work. Some cluster feed at night and express their milk during the day. Employers are increasingly accommodating the needs of nursing mothers.

In fact, it's the law in some states. Talk to your employer about creating a breastfeeding-friendly environment in your workplace.

Q: How can I tell if my baby is getting enough milk?

A: The two best indicators of adequate milk consumption are your baby's weight gain and elimination patterns. If your baby is gaining weight consistently and has between five and eight wet diapers and two to five stools per day (after the first week of life), then you are producing enough milk to nourish your baby.

Q: Doesn't breastfeeding tie you down?

A: One of the advantages of breastfeeding is mobility. You can breastfeed anywhere, and with the use of a sling, no one even knows you're doing it.

Q: How often should I feed my baby?

A: During the first week of life, you will wake your sleepy baby to nurse every two to three hours. Afterward, your baby will let you know when he's hungry. Babies typically eat eight to twelve times in a twenty-four-hour period.

Q: How can I tell if my baby is hungry?

A: Babies signal hunger by rooting (turning their mouths toward whatever touches their cheek), chewing on their fist, and making sounds. Crying is a late hunger cue. You will learn to read your baby's behavior quickly.

Q: My newborn seems to nurse all the time. Is that normal?

A: Most newborns spend an average of 187 minutes per day nursing during their first two weeks of life. It seems like a lot because they are on the breast every two to three hours, but each session lasts only fifteen to thirty minutes. Babies also tend to nurse more during growth spurts, which happen around three weeks, six weeks, three months, and six months. If your baby nurses often but doesn't wet five to eight diapers per day and have a stool at least two to five times in twenty-four hours, contact your doctor. It could be an indicator of poor milk consumption.

Q: What if I get sick and have to take medication?

A: Most medications are compatible with breastfeeding, although many doctors routinely advise temporary weaning. Talk to your pediatrician about breastfeeding-friendly medications. Pediatricians tend to be well informed on breastfeeding issues.

Q: Do I have to drink milk to make milk?

A: No. Cows don't and neither do humans.

Q: Do I have to change my diet to breastfeed?

A: Nursing mothers actually get to eat more than usual. Sometimes certain foods may cause a change in your breastmilk that upsets your baby.

Q: Will exercise make my breastmilk taste bad?

A: Ordinary exercise has not been shown to have any effect on the taste of breastmilk. However, extremely strenuous and prolonged exercise can cause a buildup of lactic acid in breastmilk, which affects the taste for about an hour.

Q: Is it healthy for my older children to watch me nurse my baby?

A: Breastfeeding is a wonderful opportunity to demonstrate breasts functioning the way nature intended. It's also the perfect time to lay the groundwork for sexual education at an age-appropriate level. Children who are raised in breastfeeding homes have a more balanced attitude regarding the human body.

Q: Is it psychologically harmful to breastfeed my toddler?

A: The benefits of breastfeeding continue as long as you nurse your child. Globally, the average age of weaning is three years. Every major health organization recognizes breastfeeding as a healthy and natural means of nurturing children of any age.

Q: Should my baby have cereal to help her sleep through the night?

A: Before six months of age, infants are unable to digest cereal. Not only will cereal upset their tummies, but it can also cause food allergies.

Q: Isn't nursing in public a form of indecent exposure? Can I be arrested?

A: No one in the United States has ever been convicted of indecent exposure for nursing in public. You have a well-established right to nurse your child anywhere you have the right to be. You are protected by law.

Appendix B

Glossary of Breastfeeding Terms

allergen: A microscopic particle of a substance that can cause an allergic reaction in someone whose immune system is sensitized.

alveoli: Small grapelike clusters of cells in the breast where milk is produced.

amenorrhea: A term for the halting of the menstrual cycle.

anesthesia: A drug administered to block pain.

antibody: Cells in the body that fight foreign cells (e.g., bacteria, fungi, and viruses).

areola: The circle of dark breast tissue surrounding the nipple.

aromatherapy: The use of scented oils, candles, or other items to influence a person's mental state.

attachment/bonding: The process of forming a strong emotional connection with another person.

baby blues: The short-term feeling of sadness resulting from hormonal imbalance and stress immediately following birth or abrupt weaning from the breast.

babywearing: The practice of carrying an infant on your body, usually in a sling.

bilirubin: A by-product of the breakdown of excess red blood cells. Extremely high levels can cause brain damage.

birth plan: An outline of your desired birthing experience.

breast abscess: An infection of the breast marked by pain, swelling, and pus.

breastfeeding: The natural act of feeding a child human milk from the mother's breasts.

breast lobes: The fifteen to twenty-five internal divisions of the breast, like the sections of an orange.

breast lobules: The twenty to forty divisions of each breast lobe that contain milk-producing cells.

breast pump: A mechanical device for expression of breastmilk.

breast shells: Domelike plastic rings used to evert nipples.

Caesarean section: Birthing in which the infant is removed surgically through the mother's abdomen.

candida: See thrush.

casein: The protein in milk that forms hard cottage cheeselike curds in the stomach.

cholecystokinin (CCK): A hormone released from the lining of the stomach that induces a feeling of satisfaction in the brain.

cleft lip/cleft palate: A condition in which an infant's lips do not grow together completely in the womb. Cleft palate refers to a similar condition affecting the roof of a child's mouth.

cluster or bunch feeding: Frequent, eager nursings with little time between sessions.

cobedding: The centuries-old practice of sleeping with your baby. Also called the family bed.

colic: A catchall term used to describe any number of conditions in babies whose symptoms include crying continuously for three or more hours, three or more times per week, for three or more weeks.

colostrum: Supermilk produced by mothers in the first few days after birthing.

demand feeding: The practice of breastfeeding a baby when she's hungry, as opposed to a predetermined schedule.

diastasis: A condition in which the vertical abdominal muscles separate during labor.

docosahexaenoic acid (DHA): An important fat that helps build brain tissue in babies.

doll-eye maneuver: Bringing your baby to an upright position so that her eyes will open, like the sleep eyes of toy dolls.

double pumping: Using a specially fitted breast pump to express milk from both breasts simultaneously.

doula: A professional labor assistant.

eczema: A skin condition characterized by dry, patchy skin.

engorgement: The enlargement of a woman's breasts caused by the onset of milk production or the buildup of milk following abrupt weaning.

estrogen: The primary female sex hormone; produced mainly in the ovaries.

evert: To make protrude; the opposite of invert.

exclusive breastfeeding: The practice of feeding a baby nothing but breastmilk.

extended nursing: Breastfeeding children who are beyond one year of age.

Family and Medical Leave Act (FMLA): FMLA entitles eligible employees to take up to twelve weeks of unpaid, job-protected leave within a twelve-month period for specified family and medical reasons.

family bed: See cobedding.

finger feeding: Allowing an infant to suckle on a clean adult finger while breastmilk is introduced into the mouth through a syringe or supplemental feeding tube.

flow rate: The speed at which milk flows through a bottle nipple.

foremilk: The first milk baby receives during a nursing session. Foremilk is low in fat and high in volume.

frenulum: The thin strip of tissue that connects the bottom of the tongue to the floor of the mouth.

galactose: One of the two sugars formed by the digestion of lactose.

galactosemia: A hereditary condition in which a child cannot digest galactose.

gastroesophageal reflux (GER): A condition in which the muscular valve at the juncture of the stomach and throat allows stomach contents and acid into the esophagus, causing a painful, heartburnlike sensation.

gavage: Feeding method in which a tube is inserted through a baby's mouth and into the stomach.

glucose: A simple sugar.

hindmilk: The breastmilk released after several minutes of nursing. Hindmilk is rich in fat and important nutrients.

hunger cues: Signals that a baby is hungry. These typically include rooting, chewing on a fist, and crying.

hypoglycemia: Low blood sugar.

hypothalamus: A part of the brain that regulates many autonomic functions like body temperature and milk production.

hypothyroidism: A condition in which the thyroid gland is underactive, resulting in many symptoms, including a diminished milk supply.

immune system: The body's protection against disease.

infant formula: Any of the artificial liquid foods designed for babies. Infant formulas are usually based on animal milk or soy.

inverted nipples: Nipples that do not protrude from the breast when stimulated.

involute: The process by which the uterus contracts following childbirth, returning to its prepregnancy size.

jaundice: A typical condition of newborns in which the child is excessively sleepy and exhibits yellowing of her skin and the whites of her eyes. Jaundice is caused by an excess of red blood cells.

kangaroo care: A style of newborn care used successfully for premature infants. The baby is placed on the mother's chest with skin-to-skin contact and ready access to the breast.

Kegel: An exercise for tightening and strengthening the muscles of the perineal floor.

Lactaid: A supplemental feeding device worn by the mother. A reservoir of milk is worn around the mother's neck and a tube from that supply is inserted into the baby's mouth as he nurses at the breast.

lactation: The medical term for the production of milk.

lactation consultant: A board-certified professional specializing in the breast and breastfeeding.

lactogenesis: The onset of milk production.

lactose: Milk sugar.

latch: The connection between baby and breast.

letdown reflex: See milk ejection reflex.

lochia: The menseslike flow of blood from the vagina following birthing.

lumpectomy: The removal of a growth or tumor without destruction of surrounding tissues.

manual expression: Removing milk from the breast using the hand.

mastectomy: Surgical removal of all or part of the breast.

mastitis: An infection of the breast characterized by flulike symptoms and swelling, redness, and tenderness of the affected breast.

mature milk: Breastmilk produced after five days postpartum.

meconium: Greenish-black, tarlike stool present in newborns.

milk bank: Storage, preparation, and distribution facilities for donated human milk.

milk ducts: The channels connecting the alveoli to the milk sinuses.

milk ejection reflex: The release of breastmilk from the milk-producing cells of the breast, caused by muscular contractions in response to oxytocin.

milk sinuses: The area beneath the areola that must be compressed to force milk through the nipple.

Montgomery glands: The small bumps on the areolas of a lactating woman that produce a substance that keeps the nipples clean and lubricated.

mylenization: The covering of nerve fibers with an insulating layer of fat.

neonatal intensive care unit (NICU): Intensive care unit for newborns such as premature infants, or others suffering from neonatal illnesses, diseases, or disorders.

nipple shields: Thin plastic protectors that fit over a mother's nipples as she nurses her child.

nursing strike: A baby's abrupt refusal to breastfeed due to some interfering factor like teething pain, a stuffy nose, or even Mom's new perfume.

orthodontic nipple: Bottle nipples that are designed to help a baby's oral cavity and teeth develop properly.

oxytocin: The hormone responsible for the milk ejection reflex.

perineum: The connective tissue between the vagina and the anus.

phenylalanine: An important amino acid.

phenylketonuria (PKU): An inherited disorder in which the body is unable to properly utilize phenylalanine.

phototherapy: The use of special lights in the treatment of newborn jaundice and seasonal affective disorder.

pituitary gland: The body's master gland, which produces many hormones, including prolactin and oxytocin.

plugged duct: A condition in which a milk duct becomes clogged, resulting in a hard spot in the breast with accompanying tenderness.

postpartum: Following labor and delivery.

postpartum depression (PPD): Feelings of despair or hopelessness following the birth of a baby and lasting longer than two weeks.

postpartum psychosis: A rare disorder of mothers characterized by hallucinations, delusions, and extreme confusion.

premature infant: A child born before thirty-six weeks' gestation.

preterm milk: Breastmilk produced by the mother of a premature infant. Preterm milk is especially high in fats, proteins, and sugars.

progesterone: Along with estrogen, progesterone is one of the two primary female hormones regulating fertility.

progestin: The synthetic version of progesterone.

prolactin: The hormone responsible for milk production.

relactating: Re-establishing breastmilk production after it has been stopped.

seasonal affective disorder (SAD): A physiological condition of depression caused by a lack of sunlight and activity. SAD is most common in northern latitudes.

sleep apnea: A condition in which a person stops breathing during sleep, often occurring many times throughout the night and requiring the sufferer to awaken in order to begin breathing again.

sleep/wake cycle: The states of consciousness and arousability. They include: quiet alert, active alert, crying, drowsiness, active sleep, and deep sleep.

sudden infant death syndrome (SIDS): Also called crib death.

supplemental feeding: Feeding done in addition to or in place of breastfeeding.

swaddling: Wrapping a baby snugly in a blanket. The practice of swaddling helps a young infant to feel secure and warm.

tandem nursing: Breastfeeding more than one child.

thrush: A yeast infection of a baby's mouth and, subsequently, the mother's nipples.

tongue thrust: The reflexive ejection of anything placed in a baby's mouth.

transitional milk: The mix of colostrum and mature milk.

weaning: The process of transitioning a child away from the breast.

wet nurse: A woman who is paid to breastfeed a child other than her own.

yeast infection: Any infection caused by yeast fungi. See thrush.

Appendix C
Resources

BREASTFEEDING INFORMATION AND SUPPORT

American Academy of Pediatrics
P.O. Box 927
Elk Grove Village, IL 60007
Tel: (847) 228-5005
Web: *www.aap.org*

International Lactation Consultants Association
1500 Sunday Drive, Suite 102
Raleigh, NC 27607
Tel: (919) 787-5181
Web: *users.erols.com/ilca/*

La Leche League International
1400 N. Meacham Rd.
Schaumburg, IL 60168-4079
Tel: (847) 519-7730
Web: *www.lalecheleague.org*

Lactation Education Resources
3621 Lido Place
Fairfax, VA 22031
Tel: (703) 691-2069
Web: *www.leron-line.com*

Mothers of Twins Clubs
P.O. Box 438
Thompsons Station, TN 37179-0438
Web: *www.nomotc.org*

Ted Greiner's Breastfeeding Web Site:
www.geocities.com/HotSprings/Spa/3156/index.html

WEB SITES

www.babycenter.com
www.babyzone.com
www.breastfeed.com
www.breastfeeding.com
www.breastfeedingresource.com
www.kidsource.com
www.naturalchild.com
www.nursingbaby.com

BREASTFEEDING EQUIPMENT AND SUPPLIES

Avent America
475 Supreme Dr.
Bensenville, IL 60106
Tel: (800) 542-8368
Web: *www.aventamerica.com*

Hollister (Ameda-Egnell)
2000 Hollister Drive
Libertyville, IL 60048
Tel: (800) 323-4060
Web: *www.hollister.com/usandcanada/*

Medela, Inc.
P.O. Box 660
McHenry, IL 60051-0660
Tel: (800) 435-8316
Web: *www.medela.com*

GOVERNMENT AGENCIES

U.S. Department of Labor
200 Constitution Avenue NW
Washington, D.C. 20210
Tel: (866) 487-2365 TTY (877) 889-5627
Web: *www.dol.gov*

U.S. Consumer Product Safety Commission
Washington, D.C. 20207
Tel: (800) 638-2772 TTY (800) 638-8270
Web: *www.cpsc.gov*

PREGNANCY AND CHILDBIRTH

American College of Nurse-Midwives
818 Connecticut Avenue, Suite 900
Washington, D.C. 20006
Tel: (202) 728-9860
Web: *www.midwife.org*

Doulas of North America (DONA)
13513 North Grove Drive
Alpine, UT 84004
Tel: (801) 756-7331
Web: *www.dona.org*

Lamaze International
1200 19th Street
Washington, D.C. 20036-2401
Tel: (800) 368-4404
Web: *www.lamaze-childbirth.com*

Web Sites

www.babiestoday.com
www.parenthoodweb.com
www.parenting.com
www.pregnancy.about.com
www.pregnancy.miningco.com

SPECIAL CONCERNS

Postpartum Depression

Depression After Delivery, Inc.
91 East Somerset Street
Raritan, NJ 08869
Tel: (800) 944-4773
Web: *www.depressionafterdelivery.com*

Postpartum Support International
927 North Kellogg Avenue
Santa Barbara, CA 93111
Tel: (805) 967-7636
Web: *www.chss.iup.edu/postpartum*

Colic

www.colichelp.com
parents.berkeley.edu/advice/babies/colic.html

Infant Massage

International Association of Infant Massage (IAIM)
P.O. Box 1045
Oak View, CA 93022
Tel: (805) 644-8524
Web: *www.lookatcyber.com/VimalaMcClure.html*

Stay-at-Home Dads

www.dadstayshome.com
www.fathering.com

Other Resources

Human Milk Banking Association of North
America
1719 East 19th Avenue
Denver, CO 80218
Tel: (303) 869-1888

University of California at San Diego Drug
Information Service
Tel: (900) 288-8273
Calls are answered 9–5, Monday through Friday. The
cost is $3 for the first minute and $2 for each
additional minute.

Books and Publications

The Art of Parenting Twins, Patricia Maxwell
Malmstrom and Janet Poland, Ballantine Books, 1999

The Breastfeeding Book, Martha Sears, R.N., and
William Sears, M.D., Little, Brown and Company,
2000

Breastfeeding, Pure and Simple, Gwen Gotsch, La
Leche League International, 2000

Caring for Your Premature Baby, Alan H. Klein,
M.D., and Jill Alison Ganon, Harpercollins
Publishers, 1999

The Everything® Baby's First Year Book, Tekla S.
Nee, Adams Media Corporation, 2002

HHS Blueprint for Action on Breastfeeding,
Department of Health and Human Services Office
on Women's Health, United States, 2000

The Nursing Mother's Companion, Kathleen
Huggins, R.N., M.S., Harvard Common Press, 1999

So that's what they're for!, Janet Tamaro, Adams
Media Corporation, 1998

Index

Page numbers in **bold** refer to illustrations.

S

School-aged children
  sexual education, 220–21
  tips for, 221–22
Separation, 265–66
Sexuality, 203
  breastfeeding and, 204
  changes in body, 211
  changing relationships, 205–6
  lack of interest, 205
  lovemaking, 103, 208–10
Shaken baby syndrome, 122
Siblings, 215–24, 288
  preschoolers, 218–20
  regressive behavior, 216, 219
  school-aged children, 220–22
  teenagers, 222–23
  toddlers, 216–18
Sickle cell anemia, 29
SIDS (Sudden Infant Death
  Syndrome), 84, 86–87
Sleep apnea, 7
Sleep chart, 81
Sleep deprivation, 193
Sleep environment, 82
Sleep/wake cycle, 79–81
Slings, 49, **49**
  colic and, 123–24
  for public breastfeeding, 142
Smoking
  around baby, 87
  complications for baby, 20–21
  milk production and, 20
  milk supply and, 192
  quitting, 20
Snacks, healthful, 181
Social preparation, 46–47
Solids
  introducing, 85, 238–39
  portions, 239

readiness for, 238
Sore nipples, 103–4
Sounds, and colic, 120–21
Soy-based formula, 170
Spitups, 74
Spoon feeding, 94, 96, 238
Stadol, 52
Standard nipples, 166, **166**
Stay-at-home dads, 259
Stay-at-home moms, 255–58
Stools, 3, 90–91
Storing breastmilk, 158–61
Street drugs, 21
Stress, 191–202
  prevention, 192–93
  relief techniques, 195–97
  support and, 200–202
Suck training, 135
Sudden Infant Death Syndrome
  (SIDS), 84, 86–87
Sudden weaning, 275–77
Sugar water, 55, 56
Supplemental feeding methods,
  94–97
Supplies, 47–52
Support
  from Dads, 202
  from family, 200–201
  from friends, 200–202
Support, lack of, 110–11
Swaddling, and colic, 123
Syringe feeding, 94, 96–97, **97**

T

Tandem nursing
  older children, 236
  positions, 132, **132**
  supplies for, 131
Taurine, 38

Teamwork, 223–24
Teen moms, and nutrition, 183
Teenagers
  sexual education, 222
  tips for, 223
Teeth, brushing, 246
Teething, 109–10, 275–76
  bottle feeding and, 173
  nipple care and, 110
Teething rings, 110
Temperament, 115–16
Thickened formula, 171–72
Thrush, 106–7
Toddlers
  moods, 218
  nursing, 232–34
  regressive behavior, 216–18
  sexual education, 217
  tips for, 217–18
Tongue thrust, 238
Tongue tie, 136–37, **138**
Tongue's frenulum, 136–37
Transitional milk, 40
Travel, 144–46
Triplets, 133
Tuberculosis, 25
Twins, 131, **132**
Tyrosine, 38

U

Urine, 90–91
Uterine contractions, 8, 41, 46,
  69, 235

V

Vegetables, introducing, 241–42
Vegetarian diet, 182–83
Vitamin supplements, 179–80

We Have EVERYTHING!

Everything® **After College Book**
$12.95, 1-55850-847-3

Everything® **American History Book**
$12.95, 1-58062-531-2

Everything® **Angels Book**
$12.95, 1-58062-398-0

Everything® **Anti-Aging Book**
$12.95, 1-58062-565-7

Everything® **Astrology Book**
$12.95, 1-58062-062-0

Everything® **Baby Names Book**
$12.95, 1-55850-655-1

Everything® **Baby Shower Book**
$12.95, 1-58062-305-0

Everything® **Baby's First Food Book**
$12.95, 1-58062-512-6

Everything® **Baby's First Year Book**
$12.95, 1-58062-581-9

Everything® **Barbeque Cookbook**
$12.95, 1-58062-316-6

Everything® **Bartender's Book**
$9.95, 1-55850-536-9

Everything® **Bedtime Story Book**
$12.95, 1-58062-147-3

Everything® **Bicycle Book**
$12.00, 1-55850-706-X

Everything® **Breastfeeding Book**
$12.95, 1-58062-582-7

Everything® **Build Your Own Home Page**
$12.95, 1-58062-339-5

Everything® **Business Planning Book**
$12.95, 1-58062-491-X

Everything® **Candlemaking Book**
$12.95, 1-58062-623-8

Everything® **Casino Gambling Book**
$12.95, 1-55850-762-0

Everything® **Cat Book**
$12.95, 1-55850-710-8

Everything® **Chocolate Cookbook**
$12.95, 1-58062-405-7

Everything® **Christmas Book**
$15.00, 1-55850-697-7

Everything® **Civil War Book**
$12.95, 1-58062-366-2

Everything® **Classical Mythology Book**
$12.95, 1-58062-653-X

Everything® **Collectibles Book**
$12.95, 1-58062-645-9

Everything® **College Survival Book**
$12.95, 1-55850-720-5

Everything® **Computer Book**
$12.95, 1-58062-401-4

Everything® **Cookbook**
$14.95, 1-58062-400-6

Everything® **Cover Letter Book**
$12.95, 1-58062-312-3

Everything® **Creative Writing Book**
$12.95, 1-58062-647-5

Everything® **Crossword and Puzzle Book**
$12.95, 1-55850-764-7

Everything® **Dating Book**
$12.95, 1-58062-185-6

Everything® **Dessert Book**
$12.95, 1-55850-717-5

Everything® **Digital Photography Book**
$12.95, 1-58062-574-6

Everything® **Dog Book**
$12.95, 1-58062-144-9

Everything® **Dreams Book**
$12.95, 1-55850-806-6

Everything® **Etiquette Book**
$12.95, 1-55850-807-4

Everything® **Fairy Tales Book**
$12.95, 1-58062-546-0

Everything® **Family Tree Book**
$12.95, 1-55850-763-9

Everything® **Feng Shui Book**
$12.95, 1-58062-587-8

Everything® **Fly-Fishing Book**
$12.95, 1-58062-148-1

Everything® **Games Book**
$12.95, 1-55850-643-8

Everything® **Get-A-Job Book**
$12.95, 1-58062-223-2

Everything® **Get Out of Debt Book**
$12.95, 1-58062-588-6

Everything® **Get Published Book**
$12.95, 1-58062-315-8

Everything® **Get Ready for Baby Book**
$12.95, 1-55850-844-9

Everything® **Get Rich Book**
$12.95, 1-58062-670-X

Everything® **Ghost Book**
$12.95, 1-58062-533-9

Everything® **Golf Book**
$12.95, 1-55850-814-7

Everything® **Grammar and Style Book**
$12.95, 1-58062-573-8

Everything® **Guide to Las Vegas**
$12.95, 1-58062-438-3

Everything® **Guide to New England**
$12.95, 1-58062-589-4

Everything® **Guide to New York City**
$12.95, 1-58062-314-X

Everything® **Guide to Walt Disney World®, Universal Studios®, and Greater Orlando, 2nd Edition**
$12.95, 1-58062-404-9

Everything® **Guide to Washington D.C.**
$12.95, 1-58062-313-1

Everything® **Guitar Book**
$12.95, 1-58062-555-X

Everything® **Herbal Remedies Book**
$12.95, 1-58062-331-X

Everything® **Home-Based Business Book**
$12.95, 1-58062-364-6

Everything® **Homebuying Book**
$12.95, 1-58062-074-4

Everything® **Homeselling Book**
$12.95, 1-58062-304-2

Everything® **Horse Book**
$12.95, 1-58062-564-9

Everything® **Hot Careers Book**
$12.95, 1-58062-486-3

Everything® **Internet Book**
$12.95, 1-58062-073-6

Everything® **Investing Book**
$12.95, 1-58062-149-X

Everything® **Jewish Wedding Book**
$12.95, 1-55850-801-5

Everything® **Job Interview Book**
$12.95, 1-58062-493-6

Everything® **Lawn Care Book**
$12.95, 1-58062-487-1

Everything® **Leadership Book**
$12.95, 1-58062-513-4

Everything® **Learning French Book**
$12.95, 1-58062-649-1

Everything® **Learning Spanish Book**
$12.95, 1-58062-575-4

Everything® **Low-Fat High-Flavor Cookbook**
$12.95, 1-55850-802-3

Everything® **Magic Book**
$12.95, 1-58062-418-9

Everything® **Managing People Book**
$12.95, 1-58062-577-0

Everything® **Microsoft® Word 2000 Book**
$12.95, 1-58062-306-9

Everything® **Money Book**
$12.95, 1-58062-145-7

Everything® **Mother Goose Book**
$12.95, 1-58062-490-1

Everything® **Motorcycle Book**
$12.95, 1-58062-554-1

Everything® **Mutual Funds Book**
$12.95, 1-58062-419-7

Everything® **One-Pot Cookbook**
$12.95, 1-58062-186-4

Everything® **Online Business Book**
$12.95, 1-58062-320-4

Everything® **Online Genealogy Book**
$12.95, 1-58062-402-2

Everything® **Online Investing Book**
$12.95, 1-58062-338-7

Everything® **Online Job Search Book**
$12.95, 1-58062-365-4

Everything® **Organize Your Home Book**
$12.95, 1-58062-617-3

Everything® **Pasta Book**
$12.95, 1-55850-719-1

Everything® **Philosophy Book**
$12.95, 1-58062-644-0

Everything® **Playing Piano and Keyboards Book**
$12.95, 1-58062-651-3

Everything® **Pregnancy Book**
$12.95, 1-58062-146-5

Everything® **Pregnancy Organizer**
$15.00, 1-58062-336-0

Everything® **Project Management Book**
$12.95, 1-58062-583-5

Everything® **Puppy Book**
$12.95, 1-58062-576-2

Everything® **Quick Meals Cookbook**
$12.95, 1-58062-488-X

Everything® **Resume Book**
$12.95, 1-58062-311-5

Everything® **Romance Book**
$12.95, 1-58062-566-5

Everything® **Running Book**
$12.95, 1-58062-618-1

Everything® **Sailing Book, 2nd Edition**
$12.95, 1-58062-671-8

Everything® **Saints Book**
$12.95, 1-58062-534-7

Everything® **Selling Book**
$12.95, 1-58062-319-0

Everything® **Shakespeare Book**
$12.95, 1-58062-591-6

Everything® **Spells and Charms Book**
$12.95, 1-58062-532-0

Everything® **Start Your Own Business Book**
$12.95, 1-58062-650-5

Everything® **Stress Management Book**
$12.95, 1-58062-578-9

Everything® **Study Book**
$12.95, 1-55850-615-2

Everything® **Tai Chi and QiGong Book**
$12.95, 1-58062-646-7

Everything® **Tall Tales, Legends, and Outrageous Lies Book**
$12.95, 1-58062-514-2

Everything® **Tarot Book**
$12.95, 1-58062-191-0

Everything® **Time Management Book**
$12.95, 1-58062-492-8

Everything® **Toasts Book**
$12.95, 1-58062-189-9

Everything® **Toddler Book**
$12.95, 1-58062-592-4

Everything® **Total Fitness Book**
$12.95, 1-58062-318-2

Everything® **Trivia Book**
$12.95, 1-58062-143-0

Everything® **Tropical Fish Book**
$12.95, 1-58062-343-3

Everything® **Vegetarian Cookbook**
$12.95, 1-58062-640-8

Everything® **Vitamins, Minerals, and Nutritional Supplements Book**
$12.95, 1-58062-496-0

Everything® **Wedding Book, 2nd Edition**
$12.95, 1-58062-190-2

Everything® **Wedding Checklist**
$7.95, 1-58062-456-1

Everything® **Wedding Etiquette Book**
$7.95, 1-58062-454-5

Everything® **Wedding Organizer**
$15.00, 1-55850-828-7

Everything® **Wedding Shower Book**
$7.95, 1-58062-188-0

Everything® **Wedding Vows Book**
$7.95, 1-58062-455-3

Everything® **Weight Training Book**
$12.95, 1-58062-593-2

Everything® **Wine Book**
$12.95, 1-55850-808-2

Everything® **World War II Book**
$12.95, 1-58062-572-X

Everything® **World's Religions Book**
$12.95, 1-58062-648-3

Everything® **Yoga Book**
$12.95, 1-58062-594-0

Visit us at everything.com

Everything® is a registered trademark of Adams Media Corporation.

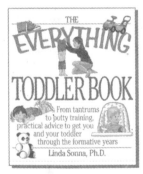